a LANGE medical book

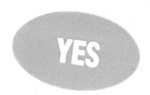

# Medical
# Epidemiology

**First Edition**

Edited by

**Raymond S. Greenberg, MD, PhD**
Professor and Dean
Emory University School of Public Health
Atlanta

*with*

**Stephen R. Daniels, MD, PhD**
Professor
University of Cincinnati College of Medicine
Cincinnati

**Dana Flanders, MD, DSc**
Professor
Emory University School of Public Health

**John William Eley, MD, MPH**
Assistant Professor
Emory University School of Medicine and Public
   Health

**John R. Boring, III, PhD**
Professor
Emory University School of Public Health

## APPLETON & LANGE
Norwalk, Connecticut

0-8385-6204-3

Notice: The author and the publisher of this volume have taken care that the
information and recommendations contained herein are accurate and compatible
with the standards generally accepted at the time of publication. Nevertheless,
it is difficult to ensure that all the information given is entirely accurate
for all circumstances. The publisher disclaims any liability, loss, or damage
incurred as a consequence, directly or indirectly, of the use and application
of any of the contents of this volume.

93 94 95 96 97 / 10 9 8 7 6 5 4 3 2 1

Prentice Hall International (UK) Limited, *London*
Prentice Hall of Australia Pty. Limited, *Sydney*
Prentice Hall Canada, Inc., *Toronto*
Prentice Hall Hispanoamericana, S.A., *Mexico*
Prentice Hall of India Private Limited, *New Delhi*
Prentice Hall of Japan, Inc., *Tokyo*
Simon & Schuster Asia Pte. Ltd., *Tokyo*
Editora Prentice Hall do Brasil Ltda., *Rio de Janeiro*
Prentice Hall, *Englewood Cliffs, New Jersey*

ISBN: 0-8385-6204-3
ISSN: 1064-1025

PRINTED IN THE UNITED STATES OF AMERICA

*In loving memory of*
*Bernard George Greenberg,*
*father, teacher, leader, and scholar.*

# Table of Contents

# Preface

*Medical Epidemiology* introduces the principles and methods of epidemiology. Although this text is written primarily with the needs of medical students in mind, students of other health professions such as nursing, dentistry, pharmacy, and veterinary medicine should find it suitable for their needs as well. Epidemiology often is taught in conjunction with biostatistics, and this book is designed to complement *Basic and Clinical Biostatistics* (Dawson-Saunders and Trapp, 1990). References to the Dawson-Saunders text are provided throughout *Medical Epidemiology* in order to facilitate using these two books together. The reader who is interested in a more focused introduction to epidemiology should find the present work to be a self-contained, independent reference, however.

## OBJECTIVES

The aim of this book is to provide the reader with an appreciation for the role of epidemiology in medicine. The authors have emphasized how epidemiology can be used to achieve the following objectives:

- Measure disease frequency
- Describe patterns of disease occurrence
- Investigate disease outbreaks
- Assess diagnostic test accuracy
- Evaluate treatment effectiveness
- Identify causes of disease development
- Predict disease prognosis

Upon completion of this book, the reader should be able to calculate and interpret basic epidemiologic measures, recognize the strengths and limitations of various study designs, understand the concepts of variability and bias, and critique published epidemiologic studies.

## APPROACH & FEATURES

The guiding prinicple in the development of this book is the presentation of epidemiology in a manner that is both understandable and interesting to the reader. This text incorporates the following features:

- The scope of topics is limited to core principles and concepts, thus reducing the overall length of the text.
- Attention is devoted to both the descriptive and comparative roles of epidemiology. In contrast to most other introductory books, chapters are included on medical surveillance and investigation of disease outbreaks.
- Each chapter begins with a Patient Profile—a clinical vignette that helps relate the epidemiologic topic to the practice of medicine.
- Data and references are drawn from up-to-date sources, thus emphasizing relevance to current applications.
- Clinical examples are drawn from content areas such as cancer, ischemic heart disease, infectious diseases, and perinatal disorders, thereby demonstrating the diverse settings in which epidemiologic methods can be employed.

- Only essential formulas and equations are included in the text with illustrative calculations. Where appropriate, more complicated mathematical relationships are described in appendices.
- Figures are used extensively in order to promote comprehension and retention of the material.
- Important concepts and principles are highlighted for emphasis.
- A summary of essential information is provided at the end of each chapter for the benefit of the reader.
- Each chapter is followed by a set of multiple-choice questions in standardized test format to facilitate self-assessment and preparation for examinations.
- An integrative chapter on the critical review of published medical literature is included.
- A glossary is provided as a guide to the correct use of epidemiologic terminology.

The authors, all of whom are practicing epidemiologists and medical educators, have attempted to infuse the text with the excitement of discovery that epidemiology has brought to their lives. To the extent that the reader is engaged by a similar sense of discovery, this book will have been faithful to its subject.

Atlanta, Georgia                                          Raymond S. Greenberg, MD, PhD
October, 1992

# Acknowledgments

Many individuals contributed to the development of this book. Alexander Kugushev, president and publisher of Lange Medical Publications, first approached the authors about writing an epidemiology text for medical students. Alex had a clear sense of the type of book that was needed, and his insights helped to shape the original prospectus and content outline. The writing began in earnest the following year, with guidance from medical editor Ruth Weinberg. Subsequently, editor-in-chief Martin Wonsiewicz oversaw the completion of the writing and helped to expedite the production process. The final art was rendered by Hal Keith, under the expert supervision of art production coordinator Becky Hainz-Baxter. Above all, a special debt of gratitude is owed to developmental editors Martha Cushman and James Ransom, who approached this project with dedication. They polished the text, detecting a variety of errors and smoothing over patches of rough prose.

Many publishers and authors kindly allowed their work to be cited in this book. Several sources of current data were particularly useful and warrant special acknowledgment: the *Morbidity and Mortality Weekly Report* of the Centers for Disease Control (Editor, Dr. Richard Goodman); the *Cancer Statistics Review* of the Surveillance Program of the National Cancer Institute (Director, Dr. Benjamin Hankey); and the *Monthly Vital Statistics Report* of the National Center for Health Statistics (Director, Dr. Manning Feinleib). The authors are grateful to J. Virgil Peavy, MS, who provided information and data about the disease outbreak described in Chapter 5.

The comments and suggestions of several anonymous reviewers were helpful in refining the style and contents of this book. In addition, Dr. Beth Dawson-Saunders and Dr. Paul Levy provided valuable advice in the developmental process. The didactic approach used in this book was developed largely through the experience of teaching epidemiology to medical students at Emory University and the University of Cincinnati. We have learned a great deal from these students and hope that their suggestions are adequately represented in the pages that follow.

The authors have had the good fortune to study under and work with a number of outstanding epidemiologists. In writing an introductory text, we were inevitably drawn back to the teachers that first attracted us to the field. The influences of former mentors can be found throughout this book. Of particular note are the teachings of Dr. Philip Cole at the School of Public Health of the University of Alabama-Birmingham, Dr. Kenneth Rothman at Boston University, and Dr. David Kleinbaum and Dean Michel Ibrahim at the School of Public Health of the University of North Carolina.

The support and encouragement of our respective institutions was essential for the completion of this project. In particular, we thank Dean Jeffrey Houpt of the Emory University School of Medicine for promoting strong educational and research linkages with the faculty of the School of Public Health. Dr. Charles Hatcher, Jr., Vice President for Health Affairs at Emory University, provided the resources and environment necessary for epidemiology and public health to develop at this institution. We also thank Emory University President James T. Laney for his vision of the role of public health in serving human needs.

Ms. Essie Mills spent many long hours in the preparation of the manuscript. For her extraordinary tolerance in dealing with countless revisions, erratic work schedules, and urgent deadlines, the authors will remain forever in her debt.

This book could not have been completed without the understanding and support of our wives and families. Time and again, precious hours at home were preempted by writing tasks, and we are grateful for the sacrifices that were made by our loved ones. Special thanks to Leah Greenberg for her advice, encouragement, love and devotion.

# Authors

**John R. Boring, III, PhD**
Professor and Director, Division of Epidemiology, Emory University School of Public Health, Atlanta; formerly Epidemic Intelligence Service Officer, Centers for Disease Control, Atlanta.

**Stephen R. Daniels, MD, PhD**
Associate Professor of Pediatrics and Environmental Health, University of Cincinnati College of Medicine, Cincinnati.

**John William Eley, MD, MPH**
Assistant Professor, Winship Cancer Center, and Senior Associate, Adjunct Faculty, Emory University School of Medicine, Atlanta, and Adjunct Assistant Professor, Emory University School of Public Health, Atlanta.

**W. Dana Flanders, MD, DSc, MPH**
Associate Professor, Emory University School of Public Health, Atlanta.

**Raymond S. Greenberg, MD, PhD**
Professor and Dean, Emory University School of Public Health, Atlanta.

# Introduction to Epidemiology

## PATIENT PROFILE

*A 29-year-old previously healthy man was referred to the University of California at Los Angeles (UCLA) Medical Center with a history of fever, fatigue, lymph node enlargement, and weight loss of almost 25 lb over the preceding 8 months. He had a temperature of 39.5 °C, appeared physically wasted, and had swollen lymph nodes. Laboratory evaluation revealed a depressed level of peripheral blood lymphocytes. The patient suffered from simultaneous infections in-volving* Candida albicans *in his upper digestive tract,* cytomegalovirus *in his urinary tract, and* Pneumocystis carinii *in his lungs. Although antibiotic therapy was administered, the patient remained chronically ill.*

## INTRODUCTION

Epidemiology is a basic medical science that focuses on the distribution and determinants of disease frequency in human populations. Specifically, epidemiologists examine patterns of illness in groups of people and then try to learn why certain individuals develop a particular disease whereas other persons do not.

Knowledge about who is likely to develop a particular condition and under what circumstances is central to the daily practice of medicine. In order to prevent an illness, health care providers must be able to identify persons who are at "high risk" and then intervene to reduce that risk. This type of knowledge emerges in many cases from epidemiologic research.

This book serves as an introduction to epidemiologic methods and the ways in which they can be used to answer key medical questions. This chapter begins with consideration of a single disease, as described in the Patient Profile. Confining our attention to this one disease enables us to demonstrate the important contribution of epidemiology to current knowledge about this condition. While the focus here is on a single disease entity, it must be emphasized that epidemiologic methods can be applied to a wide spectrum of conditions ranging from acute infectious diseases to chronic conditions such as cancer and heart disease.

The man in the Patient Profile was referred to the UCLA Medical Center in June, 1981. At the time, there was no obvious explanation why a healthy young man would suddenly develop concurrent infections of three different organ systems involving three different microorganisms. More surprising still was the nature of the infections that were present. In particular, the parasite *P carinii* was known to cause illness only in persons with impaired immune responses. The young man described in the Patient Profile, however, did not have any obvious underlying causes of immune dysfunction. For example, he did not have cancer, severe malnutrition, and he did not use immune-suppressing drugs. Why then was his body overwhelmed by the infections? This question was given a heightened sense of urgency by the severity of the patient's illness.

This patient was not the first to be referred to the UCLA Medical Center with this clinical presentation. Three other patients had been examined within the preceding 6 months, all of them previously healthy young men with recent histories of weight loss, fever, and lymph node enlargement. All had *P carinii* pneumonia and *C albicans* infections.

Why were four such patients appearing at about the same time in the same location? Suspicious that the illnesses in these four patients might be related in some way, the UCLA physicians notified public health officials and prepared a descriptive report of their findings for publication.

Was this new appearance of a rare and life-threatening form of pneumonia confined to UCLA Medical Center, or were physicians elsewhere observing similar patients? If the experience at UCLA was unique, then the entire episode might be regarded as a medical curiosity—unusual, but not a reason for great public health concern. On the other hand, if patients similar to those at UCLA were turning up in clinics or medical offices elsewhere, this episode could not be easily dismissed. Within a matter of weeks, public health authorities received reports of outbreaks of *P carinii* pneumonia among previously healthy young men in San Francisco and New York City.

In the United States, the federal agency that is responsible for monitoring unusual patterns of disease occurrence is the Centers for Disease Control (CDC).

*principle/belief*

Recognizing the potential for widespread emergence of this new, unexplained, and debilitating condition, the CDC established a special task force to collect more detailed information on the affected persons. In addition, a formal request to report such patients was issued by the CDC to all state health departments. Between June and November, 1981, a total of 76 instances of *P carinii* pneumonia were identified in persons who did not have known predisposing illnesses and were not taking immune-suppressing medications. A few months later, the disease that afflicted these patients was named the acquired immune deficiency syndrome (AIDS).

## PERSON, PLACE, AND TIME

The UCLA physicians played a crucial role in establishing the presence of a new disease in their community. The story of the first few AIDS patients—also called "sentinel cases"—is particularly dramatic because of the severity of the illness and the extent and speed with which the disease spread to affect others. In 1981, no one could have predicted that more than 150,000 persons in the United States would be diagnosed with this syndrome during the following decade. Over that same period, more than 100,000 deaths from AIDS would be reported. By 1990, AIDS had become the second most common cause of death—after accidental trauma—among men aged 25–44 in the United States.

Looking back to 1981, it is instructive to consider the features of the sentinel cases that suggested a possible connection between them. All the AIDS patients who presented to the UCLA clinicians suffered from the same rare opportunistic infections. Had the infections involved more conventional human pathogens—or less severe symptoms—then the entire episode might have gone unnoticed for some time.

Beyond their clinical similarities, the sentinel cases shared other features, as summarized in Table 1–1. All four patients were previously healthy homosexual men in their early 30s (personal characteristics) who resided in Los Angeles (place) and first became ill in the 9 months ending in June, 1981 (time). These three

**Table 1–1.** Characteristics of sentinel cases of AIDS in Los Angeles, 1981.

| Characteristic | Sentinel Cases |
|---|---|
| **Personal attributes** | |
| Age | Early 30s |
| Gender | Male |
| Prior health | Good |
| Sexual preference | Homosexual |
| **Place of occurrence** | Los Angeles |
| **Time of occurrence** | October, 1980 to June, 1981 |

dimensions—**person, place,** and **time**—are the features traditionally used to characterize patterns of disease occurrence, as discussed in Chapter 3.

## THE EPIDEMIOLOGIC APPROACH

Epidemiology is concerned with the distribution and determinants of disease frequency in human populations. Interest in disease frequency or occurrence derives largely from a basic tenet of epidemiology, ie, that disease does not develop at random. In essence, this means that all persons are not equally likely to develop a particular disease. Certain persons are at comparatively high risk by virtue of their personal characteristics and environment.

As applied to the outbreak of AIDS, for instance, it would have been highly unlikely that each of the first four identified patients in Los Angeles would have occurred in homosexual males if the disease was striking at random. The repeated occurrence of AIDS in homosexual men suggested that this segment of the population had an increased risk of AIDS. Other high-risk groups for AIDS were identified soon thereafter, including hemophiliacs and intravenous drug users. On the surface, these three subgroups may seem to have little in common. Only upon closer examination does it become evident that they all have an increased risk of exposure to the blood of other persons.

Most contemporary medical research is devoted to investigating the biologic elements of disease development. For example, in the study of AIDS, a microbiologist tends to focus on the infectious agent, human immunodeficiency virus type 1 (HIV-1), and an immunologist concentrates on the mechanisms of immune dysfunction. The epidemiologist, on the other hand, views a disease from both a biologic and a social perspective. It is not enough to know that HIV-1 is transmitted primarily through contaminated blood. The epidemiologist must be able to understand the circumstances of HIV-1 transmission among humans. Here, the influence of social factors is undeniable. One cannot fully appreciate the spread of AIDS in human populations without recognizing the role of certain behaviors, such as sexual practices or intravenous drug use.

The desire to study social factors that impinge upon health has definite implications for how epidemiologic research is conducted. In most instances, this research involves observations of phenomena that occur naturally within human populations. Such an approach is unique among the medical sciences. The features that distinguish the epidemiologic approach are (1) the focus on human populations and (2) a heavy reliance on nonexperimental observations.

At first thought, the focus on human populations may not seem at all distinctive. Ultimately, all medi-

*have an effect on*

cal research is motivated by a desire to prevent or control human illnesses. The process leading to that goal, however, may take a variety of different routes. Laboratory scientists, for example, often rely upon experiments that involve nonhuman animals or in vitro preparations. While these studies offer important advantages to the investigator, such as precise control over the experimental conditions, certain limitations must also be recognized. Obviously, a laboratory environment may not accurately reflect the actual conditions of exposure in the external world. Of equal importance is the recognition that animals of different species may have dissimilar responses to experimental manipulations. One cannot assume, for example, that biologic effects detected in rodents will necessarily apply to humans.

Epidemiologists avoid these concerns by attempting to study people directly in their natural environments. With this approach, one does not need to make assumptions about similarity of effects either across species or across doses and routes of exposure. The epidemiologist actually observes the patterns of exposure and disease development as they naturally occur within human populations. Without such information, one could never reach a definitive conclusion about the amount of disease related to a particular agent.

As with any scientific method, the epidemiologic approach has inherent constraints. In observational research, which comprises much of epidemiology, the investigator merely watches the phenomena under study. That is, the epidemiologist has no control over the events that occur. It is often difficult, therefore, to sort out the effect of interest from other background influences in the population. Even direct measurement of the degree of exposure may not be possible in some settings, thereby forcing the epidemiologist to rely upon indirect estimates.

The epidemiologist's perspective of effects in populations may appear rather crude in comparison to research at the molecular level. Indeed, epidemiology has limited utility for characterizing the precise biologic mechanisms of disease development. More often than not, the epidemiologist sees only the net effect of different levels of exposure upon the likelihood of disease acquisition.

One must realize, however, that medical progress can be achieved even in the absence of a detailed understanding of mechanisms of causation. For example, it is not necessary to characterize the molecular properties of HIV-1 in order to recognize that AIDS is a contagious disease that is spread through certain interpersonal behaviors. One can even recommend measures to prevent the spread of AIDS by reducing the frequency of high-risk practices, such as sharing of needles among intravenous drug users, without precise characterization of the infectious agent involved.

## THE APPLICATIONS OF EPIDEMIOLOGY

Epidemiologic methods can be used for a number of distinct purposes. In the following sections, these areas of application are specified, with corresponding illustrations drawn from the literature on AIDS.

### Disease Surveillance

One of the most basic questions that can be posed about a disease is the frequency with which it occurs. In order to address this question, one must know both the number of persons who acquire the disease (cases) over a specified period of time and the size of the unaffected population. Measures of disease frequency are described in Chapter 2, with application to characterization of patterns of disease occurrence in Chapter 3 and medical surveillance in Chapter 4.

The criteria used to define the occurrence of a disease typically depend on the state of knowledge about the disease and may become more refined as the causes of a disease are delineated and new diagnostic tests are introduced. For example, in 1982, the CDC created an initial, relatively simple surveillance definition for AIDS:

> A disease, at least moderately indicative of a defect in cell-mediated immunity, occurring in a person with no known cause for diminished resistance to that disease.

When the causative agent, HIV-1, was identified and tests for the detection of antibodies to the virus were developed, the definition of AIDS was refined in 1985 and again in 1987. The revised criteria allowed a diagnosis of AIDS to be made for patients with specific clinical manifestations that occur in conjunction with a positive antibody test for HIV-1 infection.

Such changes in diagnostic criteria can have a profound effect on the apparent frequency of a disease. The expanded definition of AIDS introduced in 1987 increased the number of reported AIDS patients by about 50% during the next 2 years. Accordingly, analysis of trends in occurrence over time must account for the effect of changes in disease definition.

The identification of patients with a disease can occur through a variety of mechanisms, most commonly by physician and laboratory reporting. In the United States, a number of diseases, including AIDS, must be reported to public health authorities. Collection of this information serves mainly to identify unusual patterns of occurrence. A rapid and dramatic increase in the frequency of a disease within a particular population is referred to as an **epidemic.** Early recognition of an epidemic may draw attention to the problem and help to define features of high-risk groups.

The size of the source population out of which cases arise usually is estimated for surveillance purposes from census data. The frequency of disease occurrence is then expressed as the number of new cases developing within a specified time among a standard number of unaffected individuals. For example, in the United States between February 1990 and January 1991, 16.4 cases of AIDS were reported for every 100,000 persons. This measure of the rapidity of disease occurrence is referred to as an **incidence rate.** More information on incidence rates is presented in Chapter 2.

In order to characterize patterns of disease occurrence, incidence rates may be determined for subgroups defined by geographic area. For example, incidence rates for AIDS are presented by place of residence in the United States in Figure 1–1. During this 1-year period, the incidence rate for the District of Columbia was the highest observed, with 115.7 cases for every 100,000 residents. At the other extreme, North Dakota experienced the lowest incidence rate (0.3 per 100,000). In other words, AIDS occurred in the District of Columbia almost four hundred times more frequently than in North Dakota (115.7/0.3 = 386). Why are persons in the District of Columbia so frequently diagnosed with AIDS, and, conversely, why are North Dakotans so infrequently affected?

Answers to such questions typically do not derive from surveillance information alone. Surveillance data usually are limited to general characteristics of affected persons, such as their age, race, gender, and place of residence. While variations in incidence rates according to these demographic features can lead to the identification of high-risk groups, explanations of these patterns generally call for more in-depth investigation into personal characteristics, behaviors, and environments.

## Searching for Causes

In order to study personal and environmental characteristics, epidemiologists often rely upon interviews, record reviews, and laboratory examinations. Through such sources of information, a profile of characteristics that occur in conjunction with the disease can be generated. The associations between these characteristics and the occurrence of disease can occur by coincidence, by noncausal linkages to other features, or by cause-and-effect relationships. Of course, the epidemiologist is primarily interested in the last category, ie, determinants of disease development, also known as **risk factors.** Identification of risk factors can result in a better understanding of the pathways leading to disease acquisition and thereby suggest preventive strategies.

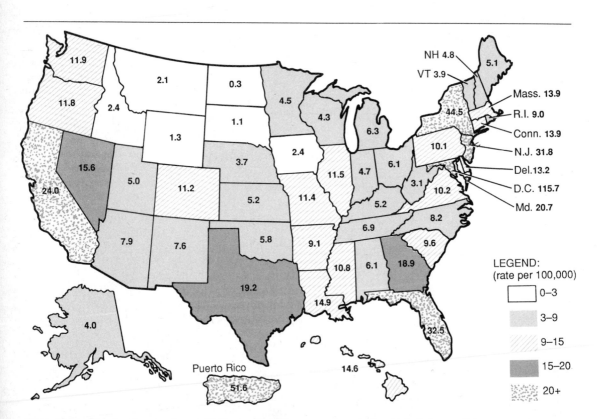

**Figure 1–1.** The incidence rates of AIDS per 100,000 person-years in the United States, February 1990 through January 1991 (Modified and reproduced from CDC: HIV/AIDS Surveillance Report, February 1991:3.)

Again, returning to the AIDS example, early epidemiologic studies played an important role in determining the cause of this disease. Within the first 5 months after recognition of this syndrome, the CDC had received reports on 70 patients in four urban centers. Of these individuals, 50 homosexual male AIDS patients were interviewed as well as 120 unaffected homosexual male comparison subjects. Persons who are affected with a disease are referred to by epidemiologists as **cases,** and unaffected comparison persons are called **controls.** Comparison of the responses from cases and controls revealed that the AIDS patients had a higher number of sexual partners. This type of investigation is referred to as a **case-control study,** and the basic design of such a study is illustrated in Figure 1–2. In essence, this study is an attempt to look backward in time to identify characteristics that may have contributed to disease development. The increased number of sexual partners—as well as a greater frequency of syphilis among cases—suggested the possibility that AIDS resulted from a sexually transmitted infectious agent, later discovered to be the HIV-1 virus. Case-control studies are described in Chapter 9.

Comparison of historical exposures reported by cases and controls can provide suggestive evidence of a cause-and-effect relationship. This type of information, however, may be distorted (biased) by differing abilities of cases and controls to recall earlier exposures. Such bias could be avoided by using a **cohort study** design in which exposure is assessed among unaffected persons and subjects are then observed for subsequent development of illness. In order to collect such data, a cohort of 2507 homosexual men without antibodies to HIV-1 (seronegative) were questioned about their sexual practices and then followed for development of antibodies to HIV-1 (seroconversion). Within 6 months, 95 men (3.8%) seroconverted, and the likelihood **(risk)** of developing HIV-1 antibodies was found to be related to receptive anal intercourse. The basic design of this cohort study is illustrated schematically in Figure 1–3. Cohort studies are discussed in Chapter 8.

## Diagnostic Testing

The purpose of diagnostic testing is to obtain objective evidence of the presence or absence of a particular condition. This evidence can be obtained in order to detect disease at its earliest stages among asymptomatic persons in the general population, a process referred to as **screening.** In other circumstances, diagnostic tests are used in order to confirm a diagnosis among persons with existing signs or symptoms of illness. Ideally, a diagnostic test would cor-

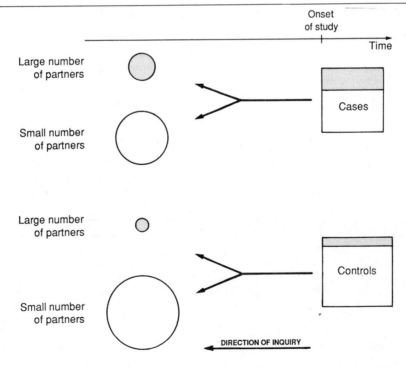

**Figure 1–2.** Schematic diagram of a case-control study of the association between the number of male sexual partners of homosexual men and the risk of AIDS. Shaded areas represent subjects with a large number of sexual partners and unshaded areas represent subjects with a small number of sexual partners.

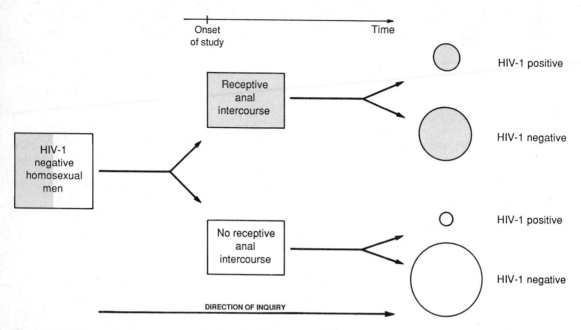

**Figure 1–3.** Schematic diagram of a cohort study of the association between receptive anal intercourse and risk of AIDS. Shaded areas indicate subjects who practice receptive anal intercourse and unshaded areas represent subjects who do not.

rectly distinguish affected persons from unaffected persons. Unfortunately, as is true of most diagnostic tests, tests for HIV-1 infection are not perfect.

Occasionally, a test will incorrectly suggest that infection is present (positive test result) in an unaffected person. This type of outcome is referred to as a **false positive,** because the positive test result was in error. Obviously, a false-positive finding for HIV-1 infection could be devastating to the tested individual, so every effort must be made to keep such mistakes to a minimum. A test with a very low percentage of false-positive results is said to have **high specificity.**

Another type of error is committed when a test incorrectly suggests that infection is not present (negative test result) in an affected person. This type of outcome is referred to as a **false negative,** because the negative test result was in error. A false-negative finding for HIV-1 infection could provide inappropriate reassurance to an infected person, thereby delaying the start of treatment and perhaps increasing the risk of spread to other persons. A test with a very low percentage of false-negative results is described as having **high sensitivity.** More detail on measures of test accuracy is presented in Chapter 6.

A number of different laboratory tests for the presence of HIV-1 infection have been introduced. The approach used most widely for screening purposes is to look for antibodies to the virus. The logic of this strategy requires two assumptions: (1) that HIV-1-infected persons have detectable antibodies, and (2)

that persons with detectable HIV-1 antibodies are infected with HIV-1. In practice, these assumptions appear to be reasonably valid among patients who are beyond the first few months of infection.

In 1985, the performance of a test for antibodies to HIV-1 was evaluated. Among 74 patients known to have AIDS with unequivocal test results, 72 (97%) had detectable antibodies. In other words, a false-negative outcome was observed for only two patients (3%). Among 261 healthy blood donors with unequivocal test results, 257 (98%) had no detectable antibodies (ie, a false-positive outcome was found for four persons [2%]). Even with highly accurate tests such as the assay for HIV-1 antibodies, interpretation of results must account for the possibility of an incorrect diagnosis.

## Determining the Natural History

In the clinical setting, one of the questions that patients ask most frequently is, "What will happen to me?" This question cannot be answered with certainty, because such predictions always involve an element of the unknown. Usually, the best guidance for predictions is the experience of other patients. Even when the ultimate outcome can be predicted with some confidence, the actual sequence of events can vary widely among patients.

Consider, for example, the situation of a patient newly diagnosed as having AIDS. In this case, the chances for recovery are virtually nil, so concern focuses on the anticipated duration of survival. In attempting to address this question, the physician might consult published research on the progression of AIDS. Usually these data are collected on large groups of patients. By noting the timing of critical events for each patient (eg, dates of diagnosis, development of further manifestations, and death), the progression of disease can be subdivided into phases. When summarized over many patients, precise and accurate estimates of the typical sequence of events—ie, the natural history of the illness—can be constructed. Some authors restrict the use of the descriptor "natural" to situations in which medical treatment is not available or is ineffective. Others use the term more broadly to indicate the typical course of an illness regardless of whether or not it can be treated effectively.

There are several different ways that one can characterize the natural history of an illness. One simple measure is the **case fatality,** which represents the percentage of patients with a disease who die within a specified observation period. For example, among all 10,233 reported adolescent and adult AIDS patients diagnosed prior to 1985 in the United States, 9248 were known to have died before 1991. In other words, the case fatality was:

$$\frac{9248}{10,233} \times 100\% = 90.4\%$$

The approach to determining the case fatality is illustrated schematically in Figure 1–4.

Another method of characterizing the natural history of a disease is to estimate the average duration from diagnosis to death **(survival time).** As an illustration, a study was conducted of all reported AIDS patients in San Francisco who were diagnosed through May, 1984, and the patients were then followed to determine whether they had died by the end of 1985. The results were then arrayed in two different but related formats. First, the investigators ordered the survival times sequentially from shortest to longest and identified as the **median survival time** the duration that was exceeded by half of the patients. In this particular population, the median survival time was found to be 11 months. Next, the investigators estimated the percentages of subjects who survived to fixed time intervals after diagnosis. Overall, only 18% of patients remained alive at 2 years following diagnosis. With the passage of time and improvements in clinical management, the survival experience of AIDS patients has improved. Therefore, one must use caution in extrapolating historical information on survival to patients currently under care.

## Searching for Prognostic Factors

Survival analysis can be employed to identify subgroups of patients with unusually favorable (or unfavorable) clinical outcomes. Characteristics that relate to the likelihood of survival are referred to as **prognostic factors.** These factors may involve demographic characteristics. For example, the relationship between age and survival was examined among almost 6000 AIDS patients in New York City. The design of this investigation is depicted schematically in Figure 1–5. It can be seen from this diagram that the study design is similar to that of the cohort study (Figure 1–3), except that the focus is on predicting survival rather than determining risk factors for the onset of disease. In this study, younger patients with AIDS tended to survive longer than older ones. Investigators found that white race and male gender are also associated with a favorable prognosis.

The clinical signs and symptoms at presentation of an illness can also serve as prognostic factors. In the study just cited, the median survival time for AIDS patients who were diagnosed with *P carinii* pneu-

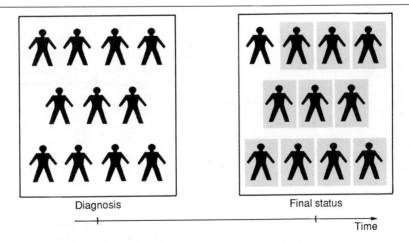

Diagnosis

Final status

Time

**Figure 1–4.** Schematic diagram of the concept of case fatality. Shaded figures represent patients who are deceased and unshaded figures represent patients who are alive.

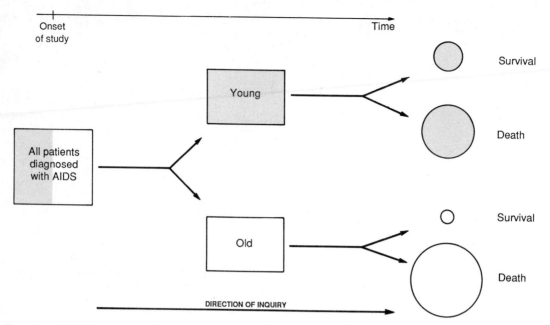

**Figure 1–5.** Schematic diagram of a study to determine whether age is a prognostic factor for AIDS patients. The shaded areas represent younger patients and the unshaded areas represent older patients.

monia alone was found to be 318 days, as compared to 750 days for AIDS patients diagnosed with Kaposi's sarcoma.

Laboratory test results also can be used as prognostic factors. For instance, derangements of blood constituents (low hematocrit and decreased levels of all white blood cells, including lymphocytes, and platelets) have been related to poor prognosis in AIDS patients. A summary of selected demographic and clinical prognostic factors for AIDS is provided in Table 1–2.

## Testing New Treatments

In the United States, all new medications must be proved effective before they can be introduced into

**Table 1–2.** Categories of selected prognostic factors for AIDS.

| Factor | Poor Prognosis Level |
|---|---|
| **Demographic features** | |
| Age | 40 years or older |
| Race | Black |
| Gender | Female |
| **Mode of presentation** | |
| Principal problem | *Pneumocystis carinii* pneumonia |
| **Laboratory tests** | |
| Hematocrit | Low |
| White blood cell count | Low |
| Lymphocyte count | Low |
| Platelet count | Low |

routine clinical care. The standard approach used to evaluate treatment effectiveness is the **randomized controlled clinical trial.** The term "controlled" means that patients who receive the new medication are compared against patients who receive either an inactive substance (placebo) or a standard treatment if there is one. "Randomized" refers to a method of treatment assignment that is determined by chance rather than patient preference or physician selection. This type of allocation system is desirable because it tends to result in study groups that are comparable with respect to important prognostic factors. Randomized controlled clinical trials are discussed in Chapter 7.

The principles of randomized controlled clinical trials can be demonstrated by a study of the effectiveness of azidothymidine (AZT) in the treatment of AIDS. AZT is a thymidine analogue with the ability to inhibit the replication of HIV-1 in laboratory tests. In early 1986, investigators at 12 medical centers in the United States enrolled 282 patients with AIDS or a related complex of symptoms in a randomized controlled clinical trial comparing AZT to a placebo. The basic design of the trial is depicted in Figure 1–6.

Randomized assignment resulted in the allocation of 145 patients to AZT and 137 to the placebo. The two study groups were similar with respect to most clinical characteristics at the onset of treatment. After an average of about 4 months of observation, the trial was terminated because of a dramatic difference in the survival experience of the two groups. Among the AZT-treated patients, only one death occurred, com-

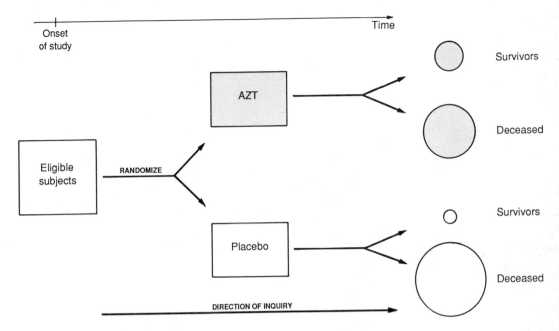

**Figure 1–6.** Schematic diagram of a randomized placebo-controlled clinical trial of AZT treatment for AIDS patients. The shaded area indicates patients randomized to receive AZT treatment.

pared to 19 deaths among the placebo-treated patients.

## SUMMARY

In this chapter, we have seen how epidemiologic research has contributed to basic knowledge about AIDS:

- The techniques of surveillance were used to determine the patterns of AIDS occurrence by person, place, and time.
- Comparisons of affected and unaffected persons led to the identification of risk factors and ultimately the suspicion that an infectious agent was responsible.
- Evaluation of tests for antibodies to HIV-1 allowed improved diagnosis and prevention of spread by contaminated blood products.
- Studies of natural history helped to define the clinical course of the illness.
- Prognostic factors were determined through comparison of patients with favorable and unfavorable outcomes.
- Finally, improvement in treatment was demonstrated through randomized controlled clinical trials.

The story of AIDS is especially dramatic because it involves a devastating disease that emerged rapidly in the population and developed with minimal advance warning. It is an unfinished story, because new cases are still occurring with alarming frequency and a cure has not yet been identified. Epidemiology will continue to play an important role in monitoring progress in prevention and treatment of AIDS.

Epidemiologic research has been pivotal in gaining insight into many different diseases. From infectious illnesses, to heart disease, to cancer, to congenital malformations, epidemiology has provided insights into patterns of disease occurrence and underlying causal factors. Ultimately, this information can be used to help control the impact of diseases either through preventive measures or improved clinical management.

## STUDY QUESTIONS

**Directions:** For each question, select the single best answer.

1. Each of the following is emphasized in epidemiologic research EXCEPT
   A. Patterns of disease development
   B. Observations of naturally occurring events
   C. Experiments with laboratory animals
   D. Characteristics associated with disease occurrence
   E. Factors that affect disease progression

2. In June and July, an outbreak of an illness occurred in a biracial southeastern state with similar sized urban and rural populations. A total of ten affected individuals were reported to the state health department by various physicians across

**Table 1–3.** Description of patients reported with fever and characteristic rash.

| Patient | Age (years) | Race | Gender | Residence | Occupation |
|---------|-------------|-------|--------|-----------|------------|
| A | 28 | White | Male | Rural | Plumber |
| B | 12 | White | Female | Urban | Student |
| C | 43 | Black | Female | Rural | Factory worker |
| D | 33 | White | Male | Rural | Farmer |
| E | 57 | Black | Male | Urban | Dentist |
| F | 69 | Black | Female | Rural | Retired |
| G | 17 | Black | Male | Rural | Student |
| H | 49 | White | Female | Rural | Secretary |
| I | 52 | White | Female | Rural | Teacher |
| J | 38 | Black | Male | Rural | Mechanic |

the state, as described in Table 1–3. Each of these individuals experienced an illness involving fever, headache, sore muscles, and a spotted rash on the palms of their hands and the soles of their feet. The characteristic that most suggested a nonrandom pattern of occurrence was:

**A.** Age
**B.** Race
**C.** Gender
**D.** Residence
**E.** Occupation

3. An epidemiologist was asked to investigate an outbreak of a respiratory illness among children attending a day care facility. Out of the 48 children at the facility, 26 developed the illness over a 2-week period. The epidemiologist plotted the days of onset as shown in Figure 1–7. The sentinel cases were indicated by the letter:

**A.** A
**B.** B
**C.** C
**D.** D
**E.** E

4. A group of 100 patients with cancer of the pancreas was followed to determine survival experience. The results are shown in Table 1–4. From these data, the estimated median survival time in months was:

**A.** 1
**B.** 3
**C.** 5
**D.** 7
**E.** 9

5. A rapid screening test for antibodies to syphilis was performed on a 19-year-old sexually active female college student who presented to the infirmary with acute abdominal pain. The antibody test result was reactive, suggesting the presence of syphilis. Further testing using a more definitive procedure indicated that the patient did not

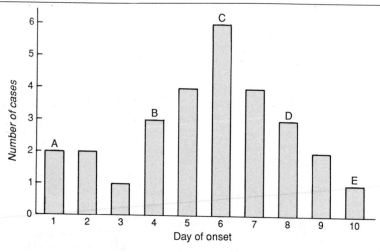

**Figure 1–7.** Distribution of patients with a respiratory illness at a day care facility, grouped by day of onset.

**Table 1–4.** Survival experience (by interval since diagnosis) of 100 patients with cancer of the pancreas.

| Interval (Time Since Diagnosis in Months) | Number Dying in Interval | Cumulative Survival at End of Interval (%) |
|---|---|---|
| 0–1 | 20 | 80 |
| 2–3 | 30 | 50 |
| 4–5 | 20 | 30 |
| 6–7 | 20 | 10 |
| 8–9 | 10 | 0 |

**Table 1–5.** Five-year survival rates for patients with stomach cancer.[1]

| Characteristic | Level | % Five-Year Survivors |
|---|---|---|
| Year of diagnosis | 1977–1980 | 17 |
| | 1981–1987 | 17 |
| Gender | Male | 16 |
| | Female | 19 |
| Race | White | 16 |
| | Black | 17 |
| Age at diagnosis (years) | 45–54 | 18 |
| | 55–64 | 16 |
| | 65–74 | 16 |
| | 75+ | 14 |
| Extent of spread | Stomach only | 58 |
| | Metastatic | 2 |

[1] Data from Ries LAG et al: *Cancer Statistics Review, 1973–88.* National Cancer Institute. NIH Publication No. 91–2789, 1991.

have syphilis, however. The original screening test was best described as:

A. True positive
B. True negative
C. False positive
D. False negative
E. None of the above

6. A 68-year-old man visited his family physician because of a persistent history of difficulty in urination. A digital rectal examination revealed that the patient had a slightly enlarged prostate with smooth contours and no evidence of masses. The patient was referred to a urologist for treatment, with a presumptive diagnosis of benign enlargement of the prostate. Surgical resection of prostatic tissue, however, revealed the presence of cancerous cells. The failure to detect the cancer upon digital examination is best described as what type of result?

A. True positive
B. True negative
C. False positive
D. False negative
E. None of the above

7. In a study of 200 patients with strokes who were treated at a university hospital and then followed to determine their clinical status 1 year after diagnosis, 120 patients had unresolved neurologic deficits and 40 patients had deaths attributed to the stroke. The 1-year case fatality in this study was:

A. 2%
B. 4%
C. 20%
D. 33%
E. 40%

8. National data on the survival experience of patients with stomach cancer are shown in Table 1–

5. From this information, the strongest prognostic factor for 5-year survival is:

A. Year of diagnosis
B. Gender
C. Race
D. Age at diagnosis
E. Extent of disease

9. Randomized controlled clinical trials are most frequently utilized to:

A. Monitor the frequency of disease occurrence
B. Identify causes of diseases
C. Improve the accuracy of diagnoses
D. Evaluate the natural history of diseases
E. Test the effectiveness of treatments

10. In a study of patients with heart attacks resulting from multiple blockages of the coronary arteries, individual patients were assigned to receive either surgical or medical management based upon the consensus recommendation of a team of cardiologists. This approach to treatment assignment was most likely to lead to a distorted comparison of surgical versus medical outcomes because:

A. No placebo group was included
B. Only two treatment options were allowed
C. The treatment groups may have differed with respect to important prognostic factors
D. The cardiologists may have disagreed on optimal treatment for individual patients
E. The number of patients in each treatment group may have differed

## FURTHER READING

Cates W Jr: Acquired immunodeficiency syndrome, sexually transmitted diseases, and epidemiology: Past lessons, present knowledge and future opportunities. Am J Epidemiol 1990;131:749.

# REFERENCES

**Patient Profile**

Gottlieb MS et al: *Pneumocystis carinii* pneumonia and mucosal candidiasis in previously healthy homosexual men. N Engl J Med 1981;305:1425.

**Introduction**

MacMahon B, Pugh TF: *Epidemiology: Principles and Methods.* Little, Brown, 1970.

**Person, Place, and Time**

CDC: Mortality attributable to HIV infection/AIDS— United States, 1981–1990. MMWR 1991;40:40.

**The Epidemiologic Approach**

Stallones RA: To advance epidemiology. Ann Rev Public Health 1980;1:69.

**Disease Surveillance**

CDC: HIV/AIDS Surveillance Report, February 1991:1.
CDC: HIV/AIDS Surveillance Report, June 1990:1.

**Searching for Causes**

Jaffe HW et al: National case-control study of Kaposi's sarcoma and *Pneumocystis carinii* pneumonia in homosexual men: Part 1, epidemiologic results. Ann Intern Med 1983;99:145.

Kingsley LA et al: Risk factors for seroconversion to human immunodeficiency virus among male homosexuals. Lancet 1987;1:345.

**Diagnostic Testing**

Weiss SH et al: Screening test for HTLV-III (AIDS agent) antibodies. JAMA 1985;253:221.

**Determining the Natural History**

Bacchetti P et al: Survival patterns of the first 500 patients with AIDS in San Francisco. J Infect Dis 1988;157:1044.
CDC: HIV/AIDS Surveillance Report, February 1991:1.

**Establishing the Prognosis**

Justice AC, Feinstein AR, Wells CK: A new prognostic staging system for the acquired immunodeficiency syndrome. N Engl J Med 1989;320:1388.
Rothenberg R et al: Survival with the acquired immunodeficiency syndrome. N Engl J Med 1987;317:1297.

**Testing New Treatments**

Fischl MA et al: The efficacy of azidothymidine (AZT) in the treatment of patients with AIDS and AIDS-related complex. N Engl J Med 1987;317:185.

# Epidemiologic Measures

# 2

## PATIENT PROFILE

*A 60-year-old male refinery worker recently developed shortness of breath and nosebleeds. On physical examination, he was pale and his pulse was elevated at 110 beats per minute. His hematocrit was 20% (low), indicating anemia, his white blood cell count was 20,000/µL (elevated), his platelet count was 15,000/µL (low), and examination of his peripheral blood smear revealed atypical myeloblasts. He was hospitalized for suspected acute myelocytic leukemia. The diagnosis was confirmed and chemotherapy was started. About three weeks after admission, the patient's temperature rose abruptly to 39° C and his granulocyte count dropped to 100/µL (abnormally low). Although no source of infection was apparent, cultures were obtained of his blood and urine, and antibiotics were administered to cover a wide range of potential infections. These cultures confirmed the presence of* Staphylococcus aureus *in the blood.*

## INTRODUCTION

The importance of risk assessment is evident in the Patient Profile. Antibiotics were administered to the patient even before an infectious cause of fever was identified. In this situation, the attending physician concluded that the potential risk of complications from delayed antibiotic treatment outweighed the likelihood of harm from treatment prior to determination of the cause of the fever. Virtually every treatment decision involves a counterbalancing of risks and benefits. In this chapter, emphasis will be placed on how epidemiologic measures can be used to assess outcomes and thereby guide decision making.

## MEASURES OF DISEASE OCCURRENCE

In this chapter, three basic measures that are used to assess the frequency of health events will be introduced. These measures, which play key roles in medicine, epidemiology, and public health, are **risk,** (the likelihood that an individual will contract a disease), **prevalence** (the amount of disease that is present already in a population), and **incidence rate** (how fast new occurrences of disease arise). In addition, these measures can be used to assess the prognosis and mortality of patients with the disease.

### Risk

Risk, or cumulative incidence, is a measure of the occurrence of new cases in the population. More precisely, *risk is the proportion of unaffected individuals who, on average, will contract the disease of interest over a specified period of time.* Risk is estimated by observing a particular population for a defined period of time, the risk period. The estimated risk ($R$) is a proportion; the numerator is the number of newly affected persons ($A$), called cases by epidemiologists, and the denominator is the size ($N$) of the unaffected population under observation:

$$R = \frac{\text{New cases}}{\text{Persons at risk}} = \frac{A}{N}$$

All members of the population, or cohort, are free of disease at the start of observation. Risk, which has no units, lies between 0 (when no new occurrences arise) and 1 (when, at the other extreme, the entire population becomes affected during the risk period). Alternatively, one can express risk as a percentage by multiplying the proportion by 100.

A hypothetical study of six subjects is presented in Figure 2–1 in order to illustrate the calculation of risk. This study began in 1982 and concluded in 1991. The time individual subjects entered the study varied, but each was free of the disease of interest at the time of enrollment. All subjects were followed for at least 2 years. For example, Patient A was enrolled in 1982, was diagnosed with the disease just prior to 1984, and then was followed until death in 1989. Patient B was enrolled in 1984, was followed until 1986 without developing the disease, and then discontinued participation in the study. Patient C was enrolled in 1986, was diagnosed with the disease just prior to 1989, and then survived through the end of observation in 1991. Patients D through F entered the study in 1984, 1989, and 1985, respectively, and each was followed through 1991 without developing the disease.

Of the six subjects under observation ($N = 6$), only one ($A = 1$) developed the disease within 2 years of

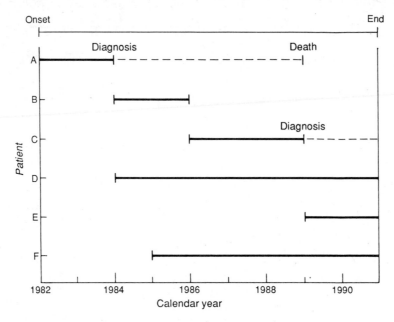

**Figure 2–1.** Hypothetical study of a group of six subjects between 1982 and 1991. The solid horizontal lines indicate time observed while the subjects are at risk for developing the disease of interest. The dashed horizontal lines indicate time observed after the subjects are diagnosed.

entry into the study. The 2-year risk of disease, therefore is estimated by:

$$R = \frac{A}{N} = \frac{1}{6} = 0.17 = 17\%$$

These same data also can be summarized as in Figure 2–2, in which the time scale on the horizontal axis represents the duration of observation for each subject. In other words, observation of a particular individual begins at time zero and continues until that person dies, is lost from the study, or the study is concluded. The format used in Figure 2–2 is sometimes preferred as a matter of convenience because it may be easier to visualize the actual relative lengths of observation of individual subjects. The following example further illustrates the use of risks and how they are estimated.

**Example 1.** In deciding whether or not to treat the patient in the Patient Profile with antibiotics prior to defining the cause of the fever, a key question facing the clinicians was, How likely is it that the patient has a bacterial infection? The answer can be based upon experience with other similar patients. In order to estimate a cancer patient's risk of acquiring an infection in the hospital (a nosocomial infection), a study was conducted of more than 5000 patients admitted to a comprehensive cancer center. These investigators carefully defined a nosocomial infection as an infection documented by cultures that was not incubating

at admission, that occurred at least 48 hours after admission, and that occurred no more than 48 hours following discharge (somewhat longer for surgical wound infections). Of the 5031 patients, 596 developed an infection that met these criteria. The risk was:

$$R = \frac{596}{5031} = 0.12 = 12\%$$

The risk period in this example for each patient began 48 hours after hospitalization and ended 48 hours after discharge. The above result indicates that about 12% of cancer patients similar to those studied would develop a nosocomial infection during or soon after hospitalization. The risk is greater than would be expected for the average hospitalized patient, suggesting that cancer patients are at unusually high risk of developing a hospital-acquired infection.

A broad range of hospitalized cancer patients were involved in this study. The man in the Patient Profile, however, had a fever and a low granulocyte count. A more refined estimate of the likelihood of infection could be derived from a study of patients with similar conditions. In one such study, 1022 cancer patients with fever and granulocytopenia were studied according to a defined protocol. Of these patients, 530 had a clinically or microbiologically documented bacterial infection. Thus, the risk of infection in granulocytopenic, febrile cancer patients is estimated to be:

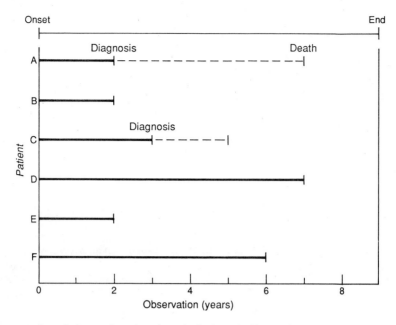

**Figure 2–2.** Restructuring of observations in a hypothetical study. Times along the horizontal axis reflect years of observation for each subject, rather than calendar years.

$$R = \frac{530}{1022} = 0.52 = 52\%$$

$$P = \frac{C}{N} = \frac{1}{4} = 0.25 = 25\%$$

This result, which suggests that the risk of a bacterial infection in patients similar to that described in the Patient Profile is very high, supports the decision to treat with antibiotics even before an infection was diagnosed.

**Prevalence**

*Prevalence indicates the number of existing cases in a population.* Specifically, the point prevalence (*P*) is the proportion of a population that has the disease of interest at a particular time, for example, on a given day. It is estimated by dividing the number of existing affected individuals, or cases (*C*), by the number of persons in the population (*N*):

$$P = \frac{C}{N}$$

Prevalence, like risk, ranges between 0 and 1 and has no units. The calculation of prevalence can be illustrated using the data summarized in Figure 2–1. For example, to calculate the prevalence of the disease of interest in 1988, two pieces of information are needed: (1) the number of persons under observation in 1988 and (2) the number of affected individuals. First, four persons are under observation in 1988 (Patients A, C, D, and F) (*N* = 4). Second, one of these persons (Patient A) is affected (*C* = 1). Thus, the prevalence in 1988 is:

**Example 2.** An important question in deciding whether or not to treat the patient described in the Patient Profile with antibiotics is the type of infection involved. A relatively small number of bacterial species cause the majority of bloodstream infections in these patients, so that therapy can be designed without definite knowledge of the actual organism involved. *Staphylococcus aureus, Pseudomonas aeruginosa, Klebsiella* species, and *Escherichia coli* account for most of the bacterial infections in these patients.

These same bacteria often can be cultured from persons without symptomatic illness. For example, the prevalence of *S aureus* skin colonization was estimated among 96 people attending an outpatient clinic for the first time. Patients with skin infections were excluded from the study. *Staphylococcus aureus* was cultured from specimens from 62 patients. The prevalence of *S aureus* colonization in this group was:

$$P = \frac{62}{96} = 0.65 = 65\%$$

From this prevalence it is estimated that in a group of patients similar to those studied, about 65% would have skin colonization by *S aureus*.

## Incidence Rate

The incidence rate (*IR*), like risk, reflects occurrence of new cases of disease. *This rate measures the rapidity with which newly diagnosed patients develop over time.* To estimate the incidence rate, one observes a population, counts the number of new cases of disease in that population (*A*), and measures the net time, called person-time (*PT*), that individuals in the population at risk for developing disease are observed. A subject at risk of disease followed for one year contributes one person-year of observation. The incidence rate is:

$$IR = \frac{A}{PT}$$

To illustrate calculation of person-time and incidence rate, consider the small hypothetical cohort illustrated schematically in Figure 2–2. Patient A developed the disease 2 years after entry into the study. Since subjects contribute person-time only while eligible to develop the disease, the person-time for Patient A was 2 years. Similarly, Patients B, C, D, E, and F contributed 2, 3, 7, 2, and 6 years, respectively. Patients A and C developed disease. Thus, *A* (the number of new cases of disease in the population) = 2, the total *PT* = 2 + 2 + 3 + 7 + 2 + 6 = 22 person-years, and the incidence rate is:

$$IR = \frac{A}{PT} = \frac{2}{22} = 0.09 \text{ cases/person-year}$$

Notice that the total person-years of observation are obtained by simple addition of the years contributed by each subject. Alternatively, this rate can be expressed as nine cases/100 person-years by multiplying the numerator and denominator by 100. Although these two expressions are equivalent, the latter might be preferred since it does not require use of decimal points.

**Example 3.** Returning to the study cited in Example 1, the incidence rate of nosocomial infections can be calculated from additional data reported in that investigation. The 5031 patients remained under observation for a total of 127,859 patient-days (or an average length of stay of 127,859/5031 = 25.4 days). Since 596 patients developed an infection that met the definition for a hospital-acquired infection, the incidence rate can be estimated as:

$$IR = \frac{596}{127,859} = 0.0047 \text{ cases/patient-day}$$

$$= 4.7 \text{ cases/1000 patient-days}$$

This means that one would expect, on average, about 0.47% of patients per day to develop a nosocomial infection among patients similar to those studied.

Calculation of incidence rates for a large population, such as that in a city, by separately enumerating the person-years at risk for each individual as described above, would require a tremendous amount of work. Fortunately, one can often calculate person-time for a large population by multiplying the average size of the population at risk by the length of time the population is observed:

**PT = (Average size of population at risk)**

**× (Length of observation)**

In many instances, relatively few people in the population develop the disease, and the population undergoes no major demographic shifts during the time period of observation. In such situations, the average size of the population at risk can be estimated by the size of the entire population, using census or other data. One can often estimate the person-time of a large stable population by:

**PT = (Size of entire population)**

**× (Length of observation)**

Example 4 illustrates calculation of incidence rates using this alternative approach to estimating person-time.

**Example 4.** In the Atlanta metropolitan area, 723 new cases of invasive cancer of the cervix occurred among white females between 1975 and 1984. An estimated 620,000 white females lived in this area on average during this time period. Thus, the woman-years of observation for this population was 620,000 women × 10 years = 6,200,000 woman-years. The average annual incidence rate of invasive cervical cancer, therefore, was:

$$IR = \frac{723}{6,200,000} \frac{\text{cases}}{\text{woman-years}}$$

$$= 0.000117 \text{ cases/woman-year}$$

$$= 11.7 \text{ cases/100,000 woman-years}$$

## DIFFERENCES BETWEEN RISK, PREVALENCE, AND INCIDENCE

As summarized in Table 2–1, incidence rates, risk, and prevalence differ in at least three important ways. First, the measures have different units. Incidence rates have units of newly diagnosed patients per unit of person-time, whereas risk and prevalence have no units. Second, these measures reflect different aspects of disease. Incidence rates and risks describe occurrence of new disease, whereas prevalence reflects already existing disease. Third, these measures are calculated differently. In Figure 2–1, the prevalence

**Table 2–1.** Characteristics of risk, prevalence, and incidence rate.

| Characteristic | Risk | Prevalence | Incidence Rate |
|---|---|---|---|
| What is measured | Probability of disease | Percent of population with disease | Rapidity of disease occurrence |
| Units | None | None | Cases/person-time |
| Time of disease diagnosis | Newly diagnosed | Existing | Newly diagnosed |
| Synonyms | Cumulative incidence | — | Incidence density |

in 1988 was 0.25, the 2-year risk was 17%, and the incidence rate was nine cases per 100 person-years. These differences imply that the three measures cannot be compared directly with one another.

In light of these inherent differences, the measures have different applications. Risks are most useful if interest centers on the probability that an individual will become ill over a specified period of time. Incidence rates are preferred if interest centers on the rapidity with which new cases arise (the time period may be long or unspecified). Prevalence is preferred if interest centers on the number of existing cases or the proportion of cases of a given type. Example 5 illustrates some of the differences between these measures.

**Example 5.** The use of an antibiotic, norfloxacin, was studied for prevention of gram-negative bacterial infections in patients with acute leukemia who had treatment-related low granulocyte counts. All 35 patients who received norfloxacin developed fever. The 35 patients were observed for a total of 220.5 person-days before first developing fever and each day, on average, about 28% of the patients had a fever. Thus, the risk of developing a fever was 35/35 = 1 in this group of patients, the incidence rate was 35/220.5 = 0.16 cases/person-day = 16 cases/100 person-days, and the average prevalence was 28%.

The risk of 1 suggests that treatment with norfloxacin does not ultimately prevent infectious fevers or reduce risk of fever development. On the other hand, the incidence rate in the norfloxacin- treated group was lower than that in a group of similar patients who did not receive norfloxacin, suggesting that treatment slowed or delayed the onset of fever. Furthermore, prevalence of fever was lower in the norfloxacin group, which indicates that treated patients are less likely to be febrile on an "average" day.

## SURVIVAL

Survival is the probability of remaining alive for a specific length of time. For a chronic disease such as cancer, 1-year survival and 5-year survival are often used as indicators of the severity of disease and the prognosis. For example, the 5-year survival for lung cancer is about 0.13, indicating that only 13% of lung cancer cases survive at least 5 years after diagnosis.

In simple situations, one estimates survival ($S$) as:

$$S = \frac{A - D}{A}$$

where $D$ is the number of deaths observed in a specified period of time and $A$ is the number of newly diagnosed patients under observation. Survival for at least 2 years after diagnosis can be determined from the data in Figure 2–3. Observation of each patient begins at diagnosis (time = 0), and continues until: death, survival for 5 years, or follow-up ceases (the subject is "censored"). A patient is censored when follow-up ends prior to death or completion of a full period of observation. Follow-up could end for one of several reasons: (1) the patient decides to discontinue participation, (2) the patient is "lost" to follow-up, or (3) the study ends. Five of the six people under observation ($N = 6$) in Figure 2–3 survive at least 2 years. Thus, the 2-year survival is:

$$S = \frac{5}{6} = 0.83 = 83\%$$

Calculation of survival indicates probability of surviving a specified length of time, and is inversely related to the risk of death. Survival estimates provide a useful way to summarize prognosis, as illustrated in Example 6.

**Example 6.** The patient described in the Patient Profile has acute myelocytic leukemia, a type of acute nonlymphocytic leukemia. Data collected by the National Cancer Institute for patients diagnosed with this disease between 1981 and 1987 in the United States indicate that only about 9% of patients survived for at least 5 years from the time of diagnosis. For persons who were under 65 years of age at diagnosis, the 5-year survival rate (14%) was higher than that for those who were 65 or older at diagnosis (2%). Nevertheless, it can be concluded from these data that, regardless of age, patients with acute myelocytic leukemia have an extremely poor prognosis.

## Life Table and Other Survival Analyses

When studying survival and risk, problems can arise if the investigator cannot follow some subjects for the entire risk period. This situation may arise if some subjects move away or miss a follow-up appointment. In Figure 2–3, for example, observation of Patients B and E stopped after 2 years (censored). If one wishes to determine the survival for a 5-year

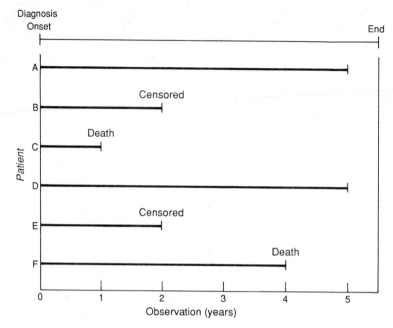

**Figure 2–3.** Survival experience of a hypothetical group of six patients. The time of observation for each subject, beginning with diagnosis, is measured in years.

period, observation of Patients B and E is incomplete. One knows only that these individuals survived for at least 2 years, not if they survived a full 5 years. Incomplete observations like these make it difficult to calculate survival. If one assumes that Patients B and E both survived the full 5 years, the survival estimate would be:

$$S = \frac{4}{6} = 0.67 = 67\%$$

On the other hand, if one assumes that neither of these patients survived for 5 years, then the survival estimate would be:

$$S = \frac{2}{6} = 0.33 = 33\%$$

Since the observations are incomplete, we do not know which, if either, of these two calculations is correct. This inability to estimate the survival probabilities with incomplete observations underscores the need for analytic methods to handle censored observations.

Statisticians have developed special techniques, called survival analyses, to account for such incomplete observations. Two particularly useful methods of survival analysis are life table analysis and Kaplan-Meier analysis. Life table and Kaplan-Meier analyses allow calculation of risks even if some of the observations are incomplete. Descriptions of these and other methods of survival analysis can be found in *Basic*

*and Clinical Biostatistics* (Dawson-Saunders and Trapp, 1990).

The results of a survival analysis can be presented graphically as shown in Figure 2–4. The information portrayed in this graph relates to the survival experience of adult patients with leukemia in the United States. Along the horizontal axis, time in years since diagnosis is plotted (0 = time of diagnosis). Along the vertical axis, the percentage of patients who are alive is plotted. The survival curve begins at the time of diagnosis, when 100% of patients are alive. During the first year following diagnosis, 40% of the patients die. During the next year, another 10% of patients die. The process of attrition to death continues through the end of the 5-year observation period.

The survival curve can be used to determine basic summary measures about the prognosis of leukemia in adults. For example, one may wish to know the percentage of patients that survive to some fixed period of time following diagnosis. Typically, cancer prognosis is assessed by determining the percentage of patients who survive for at least 5 years after diagnosis. The approach to estimating this percentage is depicted in Figure 2–5. Beginning on the horizontal axis at 5 years, a line is drawn to the survival curve (Step A). From the point of intersection with the survival curve, a line is drawn across to the vertical axis (Step B). The percentage of survivors (35%) is then read from the vertical axis.

Another summary measure of prognosis is the median survival time, which is the time following diagnosis at which one-half of the patients remain alive.

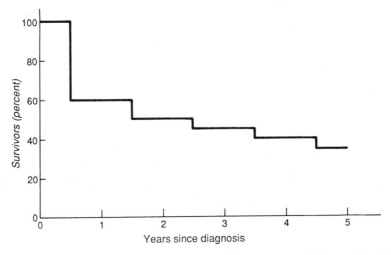

**Figure 2–4.** Survival curve for patients diagnosed with any type of leukemia in 1983 in the United States. (Data from Ries LAG et al: *Cancer Statistics Review, 1973–1988.* National Cancer Institute. NIH Publication No. 91–2789, 1991.)

The approach to estimating the median survival time is shown in Figure 2–6. Beginning on the vertical axis at the 50% (median) survival level, a line is drawn across to the survival curve (Step A). From the midpoint of intersection with the survival curve, a line is drawn down to the horizontal axis (Step B). The median survival time in this example is estimated to be 2 years.

## Case Fatality

The propensity of a disease to cause the death of affected patients is referred to as the **case fatality** (the terms "rate" and "ratio" are sometimes associated with "case fatality," although mathematically this is not appropriate). Case fatality (CF) is estimated by:

$$CF = \frac{\text{Number of deaths}}{\text{Number of diagnosed patients}} = \frac{D}{A}$$

The resulting estimate can be left as a proportion, or multiplied by 100 to convert it to a percentage. Notice that this formula is analogous in structure to that previously described for risk, or cumulative incidence. The difference between these two measures is the phase of illness to which they are applied. Risk of disease refers to the initial development of the condition, and case fatality refers to the likelihood of death from the disease. Both measures require specification of some time period over which events are counted.

The relationship between risk and case fatality is depicted schematically in Figure 2–7. The initial pop-

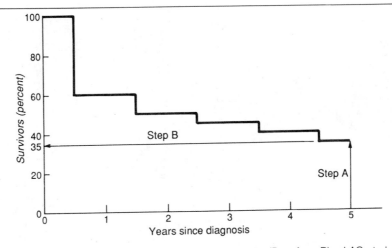

**Figure 2–5.** Approach to estimating the survival 5 years after diagnosis. (Data from Ries LAG et al: *Cancer Statistics Review, 1973–1988.* National Cancer Institute. NIH Publication No. 91–2789, 1991.)

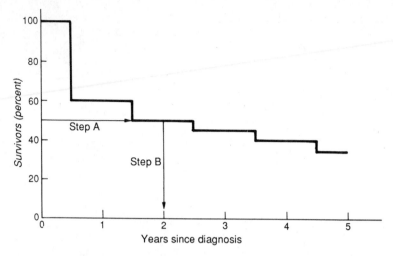

**Figure 2–6.** Approach to estimating the median survival time. (Data from Ries LAG et al: *Cancer Statistics Review, 1973–1988.* National Cancer Institute. NIH Publication No. 91–2789, 1991.)

ulation at risk of disease consists of 15 women ($N = 15$), five of whom develop the condition of interest. Risk, or cumulative incidence, therefore, is:

$$R = \frac{A}{N} = \frac{5}{15} = 0.33 = 33\%$$

Only two ($D = 2$) of the affected women ($A = 5$)

subsequently die from the condition. The case fatality, therefore, is:

$$CF = \frac{D}{A} = \frac{2}{5} = 0.40 = 40\%$$

The case fatality can range from 0, when no patients die from the disease, to 1 (or 100%), when all patients

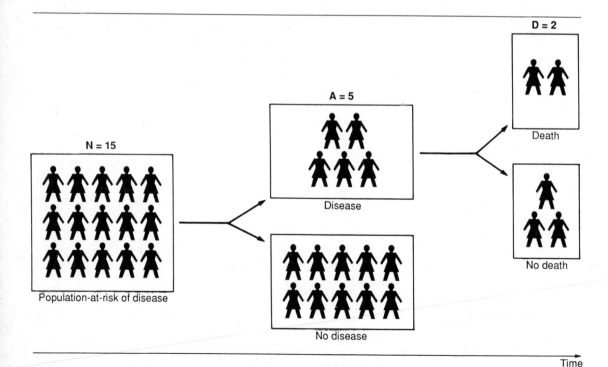

**Figure 2–7.** Schematic diagram of the natural history of an illness, indicating the population at risk of disease (N), incident cases (A), and deaths from the disease (D).

die from the disease. Since the case fatality represents the proportion of persons affected with a disease who die from it, the case fatality may be thought of as the complement to survival. In other words, for a given period of observation, the case fatality and survival should sum to 100%. Returning to Figure 2–7, survival is:

$$S = \frac{(A - D)}{A} = \frac{(5 - 2)}{5} = \frac{3}{5} = 0.60 = 60\%$$

Thus, the case fatality ($CF = 40\%$) and the survival ($S = 60\%$) total 100%.

## SUMMARY

Five of the basic descriptive measures used in epidemiology have been introduced in this chapter. Although other indicators of disease frequency and prognosis exist, these five measures are central to the descriptive function of epidemiology. Key points to remember are listed below.

(1) **Risk,** or cumulative incidence, is the proportion of unaffected persons who develop the disease of interest in a specified period of time.
(2) **Prevalence** is the number of persons affected by the disease of interest at a particular time.
(3) **Incidence rate** measures the rapidity with which unaffected persons develop a particular disease.
(4) **Survival** is the proportion of persons affected by the disease of interest who live for at least a specified period of time.
(5) **Case fatality** is the proportion of persons affected by a particular disease who die from it within a specified period of time.

Survival and case fatality represent mutually exclusive outcomes, and together must account for all individuals affected with the disease who have known vital status.

Application of these measures to the questions raised by the Patient Profile resulted in the following conclusions:

(1) Hospitalized cancer patients have a substantial risk ($R = 0.12$, or 12%) of developing an infection during hospitalization.
(2) The infectious agents that cause bloodstream infections (eg, *S aureus*) in cancer patients, are commonly cultured from the skin of healthy persons (prevalence [$P$] $= 0.65$, or 65%).
(3) The incidence rate of infection among hospitalized cancer patients is appreciable ($IR = 4.7$ cases per 1000 patient-days), but the corresponding incidence rate for patients with impaired immune systems is more than 30 times greater ($IR = 160$ cases per 1000 patient-days).

(4) The 5-year survival for adult patients with acute myelocytic leukemia is extremely low ($S = 0.09$, or 9%).
(5) Based upon the survival data, it can be concluded that over 90% of patients with acute myelocytic leukemia die from this disease, or its complications, within 5 years of diagnosis.

With this information in mind, the physician in the Patient Profile can conclude that the patient is at unusually high risk for a life-threatening nosocomial bacterial infection. Rapid initiation of antibiotic therapy is warranted even before the results of bacterial cultures are known. By appropriate use and interpretation of standard epidemiologic measures, such as risk and incidence rate, the physician can make an informed and potentially life-saving treatment decision.

## STUDY QUESTIONS

**Directions:** For each question, select the single best answer.

**Questions 1–3:** A study about risk of stroke among elderly hypertensive patients was conducted between 1986 and 1991. The results of observations on six patients are depicted graphically in Figure 2–8.

1. The prevalence of stroke among these patients in 1988 is:
   A. $1/6 = 0.17$
   B. $2/6 = 0.33$
   C. $2/5 = 0.40$
   D. $3/6 = 0.50$
   E. $3/5 = 0.60$

2. The 2-year risk of developing a stroke among these patients is:
   A. $1/6 = 0.17$
   B. $2/6 = 0.33$
   C. $2/5 = 0.40$
   D. $3/6 = 0.50$
   E. $3/5 = 0.60$

3. The 1-year survival rate following a stroke is:
   A. $1/6 = 0.17$
   B. $1/3 = 0.33$
   C. $1/2 = 0.50$
   D. $2/3 = 0.67$
   E. $3/3 = 1.0$

**Questions 4–5:** A survival curve for women with ovarian cancer is shown in Figure 2–9.

4. From this curve, the 5-year survival is estimated to be closest to:
   A. 45%
   B. 55%
   C. 65%
   D. 75%
   E. 85%

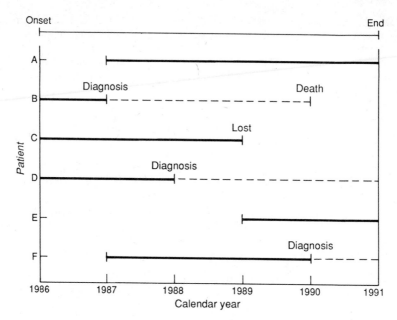

**Figure 2–8.** Observations on six elderly hypertensive patients (A–F). The solid lines indicate times observed while the subjects were at risk of developing strokes, and the dashed lines indicate times observed after strokes.

5. The median survival time in years for ovarian cancer patients is estimated to be about:
   A. 1
   B. 2
   C. 3
   D. 4
   E. 5

**Questions 6–8:** Within a population of 1000 adults, an initial clinical examination reveals 100 individuals with diabetes mellitus. Over the following 10 years, 40 additional subjects develop diabetes mellitus; five of these individuals die within 5 years of their diagnosis.

6. The initial prevalence of diabetes mellitus in this population is:
   A. 100/1000
   B. 100/900
   C. 40/1000
   D. 40/900
   E. 40/100

7. The risk of developing diabetes mellitus within 10 years is:

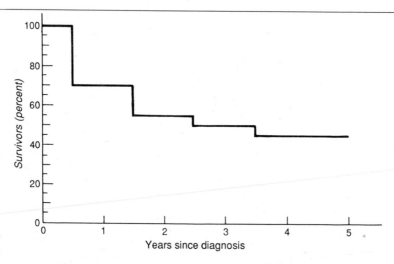

**Figure 2–9.** Survival curve for patients with ovarian cancer.

**A.** 100/1000
**B.** 100/900
**C.** 40/1000
**D.** 40/900
**E.** 40/100
8. The 5-year case fatality of the incident cases is:
**A.** 5/100
**B.** 5/40
**C.** 5/(100 + 40)
**D.** 5/900
**E.** 5/1000

**Questions 9–10:** Survival data are shown in Table 2–2 for 100 patients consecutively admitted to a burn treatment center.
9. Based on these data, survival for the first 28 days after admission is:
**A.** 1/90 = 0.01
**B.** 89/90 = 0.99
**C.** 89/95 = 0.94

Table 2–2. Data on survival experience of 100 burn patients.

| Days Since Admission | Number of Patients | | |
|---|---|---|---|
| | Total | Die | Survive |
| 1–7 | 100 | 5 | 95 |
| 8–14 | 95 | 3 | 92 |
| 15–21 | 92 | 2 | 90 |
| 22–28 | 90 | 1 | 89 |

**D.** 11/100 = 0.11
**E.** 89/100 = 0.89
10. Based upon these data, case fatality for the first 28 days after admission is:
**A.** 1/90 = 0.01
**B.** 89/90 = 0.99
**C.** 89/95 = 0.94
**D.** 11/100 = 0.11
**E.** 89/100 = 0.89

## FURTHER READING

Elandt-Johnson RC: Definition of rates: Some remarks on their use and misuse. Am J Epidem 1975;102:267.
Flanders WD, O'Brien TR: Inappropriate comparisons of incidence and prevalence in epidemiologic research. Am J Pub Health 1989;79:1301.

## REFERENCES

**Risk**
European Organization for Research and Treatment of Cancer International Antimicrobial Therapy Cooperative: Ceftazidime combined with a short or long course of amikacin for empirical therapy of gram-negative bacteremia in cancer patients with granulocytopenia. N Engl J Med 1987;317:1692.
Rotstein C et al: Nosocomial infection rates at an oncology center. Infect Control Hosp Epidemiol 1988;9:13.

**Prevalence**
Schimpff SC: Empiric antibiotic therapy for granulocytopenic cancer patients. Am J Med 1986;80:13.

**Incidence Rate**
Greenberg RS, Chow WH, Liff JM: Recent trends in the epidemiology of cervical neoplasia. Acta Cytol 1989;33:463.

**Differences Between Risk, Prevalence, and Incidence**
Karp JE et al: Oral norfloxacin for prevention of gram-negative bacterial infections in patients with acute leukemia and granulocytopenia. Ann Intern Med 1987; 106:1.

**Survival**
Ries LAG et al: *Cancer Statistics Review, 1973–88*. National Cancer Institute. NIH Publication No. 91–2789, 1991.

**Life Table and Other Survival Analyses**
Dawson-Saunders B, Trapp RG: *Basic and Clinical Biostatistics*. Appleton & Lange, 1990.
Evans C et al: High-dose cytosine arabinoside and L-asparaginase therapy for poor-risk adult acute non-lymphocytic leukemia. Cancer 1990;66:2624.

## PATIENT PROFILE

*A 32-year-old male electrician who recently immigrated to the United States from Southeast Asia came to the emergency room with a 6-week history of cough, fever, night sweats, weakness, fatigue, and shortness of breath. Cavitary lesions were visible on the patient's chest x-ray. A smear of a sputum specimen revealed acid-fast bacilli.* Mycobacterium tuberculosis *subsequently grew from cultures of the sputum, and these organisms were susceptible to all drugs tested. The patient was placed on an antibiotic regimen involving three medications. After 2 weeks of pharmacologic therapy, the patient was clinically improved and there was no evidence of bacilli in his sputum. He was instructed to continue antibiotic treatment for at least 6 months.*

*The patient resided with his wife and two young children in an apartment building. Tuberculin skin tests were administered to each of the family members, and results were positive for the patient's wife and three-year-old daughter. Although no evidence of clinically active tuberculosis was found in either the wife or daughter, preventive therapy with isoniazid was administered to all three family members. Skin testing of all 54 of the other residents of the apartment building revealed one other infected adult, who lacked evidence of active disease and received preventive antibiotic therapy. None of the tuberculin skin tests administered to the patient's coworkers were positive.*

## CLINICAL BACKGROUND

Tuberculosis is caused by bacteria that are transmitted on small airborne particles created when an individual with pulmonary tuberculosis coughs or sneezes. Air currents circulate these particles throughout an entire room or building. When a susceptible person inhales these particles, bacteria may become established in the lungs and spread throughout the body. Usually the host's immune system contains this initial infection within a short period of time. A small proportion (5–10%) of patients will develop active clinical illness months to years later when the bacteria begin to replicate and cause symptoms.

As shown in Table 3–1, environmental as well as personal factors affect the likelihood of tuberculosis transmission. Each of the environmental features listed tends to increase the concentration of bacteria in the air. Transmission also is promoted by characteristics of the infected individual that contribute to greater release of bacteria and characteristics of the susceptible person that diminish the immune response.

Public health officials in the United States have developed a strategic plan for the elimination of tuberculosis in this country by the year 2010. An effective plan for the control of tuberculosis requires that persons with active tuberculosis are identified early, while infectious, isolated from susceptible persons, and treated with adequate antibiotic therapy. Control strategies also include screening for the presence of asymptomatic infection within groups at high risk of tuberculosis, followed by antibiotic therapy to prevent the development of active disease. On the basis of epidemiologic data, a number of groups with elevated risks of tuberculosis have been identified (Table 3–2).

The Patient Profile illustrates many important points about tuberculosis. Since the patient had recently left an area with an elevated prevalence of tuberculosis, he was a member of a high-risk group. The presence of symptoms, in conjunction with cavitary lung lesions and bacilli in the sputum, indicated that the patient was highly infectious. Although the infectious state may end after several weeks of appropriate antibiotic treatment, relapse may occur unless therapy is sustained for at least 6 months.

Once a patient is diagnosed with clinically active tuberculosis, the patient's close personal contacts should be tested for tuberculosis. The wife and two children of the man in the Patient Profile were considered close contacts. Since asymptomatic infection was demonstrated in the wife and one child, preventive therapy was administered. The other child showed no signs of infection. Guidelines for preventive therapy dictate that children who are close contacts should receive antibiotics until a negative skin

**Table 3–1.** Factors that increase the probability of tuberculosis transmission.

**Environment**
  Close contact of infectious and susceptible people in small, enclosed spaces
  Poor ventilation
  Recirculation of contaminated air
**Infectious individuals**
  Pulmonary or laryngeal disease (especially with bacilli in sputum or cavitary lesions in the lung)
  Cough or other cause of forceful expiration; uncovered mouth when coughing
  Less than 2–3 weeks of appropriate antimicrobial therapy
**Susceptible individuals**
  Compromised immune system
  Presence of certain predisposing medical conditions (eg, silicosis, cancer)
  Lack of adequate nutrition
  Intravenous drug use or heavy alcohol intake

test is repeated 12 weeks later. Residents of the patient's apartment building and his coworkers also were considered to be at high risk and were investigated for infection. The single infected resident was treated with preventive antibiotics, in accordance with established guidelines.

## DESCRIPTIVE EPIDEMIOLOGY

Broadly speaking, epidemiologic work can be divided into two main categories: (1) **descriptive epidemiology,** which includes activities related to characterizing the distribution of diseases within a population, and (2) **analytic epidemiology,** which concerns activities related to identifying possible causes for the occurrence of diseases. Both types of epidemiology are fundamental to the prevention and control of diseases and to the advancement of medical knowledge. Descriptive patterns of disease occurrence often lead to hypotheses about disease causation that are tested in analytic investigations. Analytic studies may yield findings that help to explain descriptive patterns and improve surveillance efforts.

**Table 3–2.** Populations at high risk of tuberculosis.

Persons with the human immunodeficiency virus (HIV)
Family members and close personal contacts of persons with tuberculosis
Individuals with predisposing medical conditions, such as silicosis, hematologic disorders, cancer, chronic renal failure, and diabetes mellitus
Foreign-born persons from countries where the prevalence of tuberculosis is high
Medically underserved low-income populations
Alcohol and intravenous drug users
Residents of long-term facilities, such as correctional institutions, nursing homes, and mental institutions
Health care workers

The tools for descriptive epidemiology, measures of disease occurrence, were introduced in Chapter 2. In the present chapter, these tools are used to characterize the population distribution of tuberculosis. Toward that end, three basic questions can be asked:

(1) **Who** develops tuberculosis?
(2) **Where** does tuberculosis occur?
(3) **When** does tuberculosis occur?

Collectively, these three questions serve as the basis for a descriptive investigation of tuberculosis. Answers to these questions characterize the distribution of tuberculosis by **person, place,** and **time.** As shown schematically in Figure 3–1, these features are the standard dimensions used to track the occurrence of a disease.

### Person

A basic tenet of epidemiology is that diseases do not occur at random. In other words, not all persons within a population are equally likely to develop a particular condition. Variation of occurrence in relation to personal characteristics may reflect differences in level of exposure to causal factors, susceptibility to the effects of causal factors, or both exposure and susceptibility.

Typically, the personal characteristics that are examined with respect to disease occurrence are age, race, and gender. Since such information is collected routinely on the affected persons (cases), as well as the unaffected population from which the cases develop, epidemiologists rely on these characteristics to a great extent. The use of other attributes of interest, such as level of education and income, marital status, and occupation, is contingent upon the availability of data.

The distribution of cases of tuberculosis reported in the United States during 1989 is shown in Figure 3–2. From this graph, it appears that the age group with the highest risk of tuberculosis is 25 to 44 years. This conclusion is incorrect, however, because it fails to take into account the varying sizes of the source populations of the different age groups. The larger number of cases occurring between 25 and 44 years of age, as compared to those 65 years or older, is explained by the larger number of persons in the general population in the 25–44-year-old group. By calculating incidence rates, one can compensate for disparities in sizes of the source of populations. As illustrated in Figure 3–3, the incidence of tuberculosis is elevated at the extremes of age, particularly among the elderly.

A number of factors contribute to the nonrandom relationship between tuberculosis incidence and age. First, the long latent period between infection and development of clinical symptoms means that the ages at detection of illness are expected to be skewed

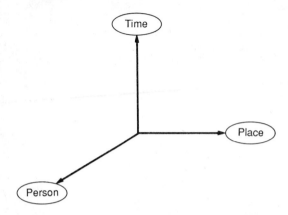

**Figure 3–1.** Schematic representation of the standard dimensions used to characterize disease occurrence.

toward later life. Second, since elderly individuals lived through time periods when the disease was more common, they are more likely to have been infected than younger persons **(birth cohort effect).** Third, older persons are more likely to have other illnesses (eg, cancer, diabetes mellitus) that may make them more susceptible to tuberculosis. Fourth, the decline in immune function associated with the normal aging process may increase susceptibility. Fifth, elderly persons are more likely to live in closed communal settings that are conducive to the spread of tuberculosis.

An equally striking nonrandom pattern of occurrence is seen when incidence is examined as a function of race or ethnicity (Figure 3–4). The highest incidence rate of tuberculosis in the United States is found among Asians and Pacific Islanders; it is almost nine times greater than the rate for white non-Hispanics. The vast majority of tuberculosis cases

among Asians and Pacific Islanders in the United States occurs among foreign-born persons. Most of these individuals, as exemplified by the subject of the Patient Profile, acquire the infection in the high-risk country of origin but do not develop symptomatic disease until they arrive in the United States. A high proportion of tuberculosis cases among Hispanics in the United States also occurs in foreign-born persons.

The high incidence rates of tuberculosis within other minority groups in the United States reflect the influences of other risk factors. Tuberculosis is a disease that is associated with socioeconomic disadvantage. The combination of crowded housing, poor nutrition, inadequate access to preventive and therapeutic medical services, alcoholism and intravenous drug use, as well as any predisposing medical conditions, contributes to the high risk of tuberculosis among the poor. Since black and Native American/Alaskan Native populations in the United States have disproportionately large numbers of disadvantaged persons, the incidence of tuberculosis in these communities is elevated.

The distribution of tuberculosis by gender is shown in Figure 3–5. The incidence of tuberculosis is twice as high among males as among females. The higher occurrence of tuberculosis among males probably is related to gender differences in certain high-risk behaviors (eg, heavy alcohol consumption), as well as predisposing diseases (eg, AIDS, silicosis).

### Place

Variation in the place of occurrence of a disease can be evaluated at the national level (eg, across countries), at the regional level (eg, across states), or at the local level (eg, across communities). Certain countries, particularly those in the nonindustrialized parts of the world, have comparatively high rates of

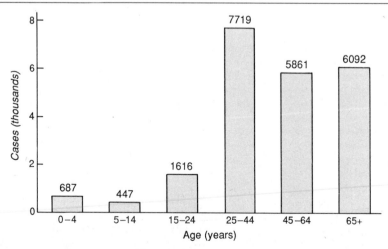

**Figure 3–2.** Number of reported cases of tuberculosis by age in the United States, 1989. (Data from CDC: Update: Tuberculosis elimination–United States. MMWR 1990;39:153.)

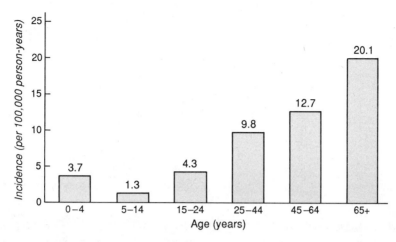

**Figure 3–3.** Incidence rates for reported tuberculosis, grouped by age, in the United States in 1989. (Data from CDC: Update: Tuberculosis elimination–United States. MMWR 1990;39:153.)

tuberculosis occurrence. The estimated incidence rates of this disease across various parts of the developing world are shown in Figure 3–6. These rates are estimates because the actual reporting of new cases is incomplete in many nonindustrialized countries. Accordingly, this information must be interpreted with caution. Even the lowest of these estimates, however, is more than ten times greater than the corresponding incidence in the United States and other industrialized countries. The high rates of tuberculosis in the nonindustrialized nations are attributable to poverty, inadequate preventive and therapeutic programs, and particularly in sub-Saharan Africa, the high prevalence of infection with human immunodeficiency virus (HIV).

Even within an industrialized country, such as the United States, variation in the incidence of tuberculosis is observed (Figure 3–7). The highest rates occur in the District of Columbia and New York State. Comparatively low rates are found in the west north central and mountain regions. These geographic patterns probably reflect demographics and predisposing conditions, such as intravenous drug use and infection with HIV.

**Time**

The overall incidence of tuberculosis between 1980 and 1989 in the United States is depicted in Figure 3–8. During the first part of the 1980s, a consistent downward trend was observed, continuing a pattern that began many decades earlier. After 1984, however, the incidence of this disease remained fairly constant. Another way to visualize this pattern is to

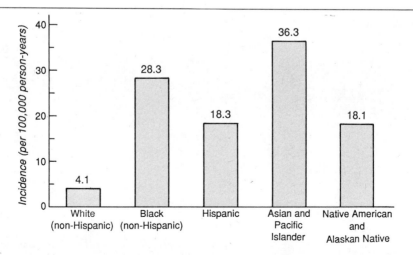

**Figure 3–4.** Incidence rates for reported tuberculosis, grouped by race/ethnicity, in the United States in 1989. (Data from CDC: Update: Tuberculosis elimination–United States. MMWR 1990;39:153.)

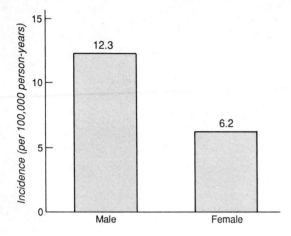

**Figure 3–5.** Incidence rates for reported tuberculosis, grouped by gender, in the United States in 1989. (Data from CDC: Update: Tuberculosis elimination–United States. MMWR 1990;39:153.)

compare the percentage change in incidence between the first and last years of 3-year time intervals (Figure 3–9). Between 1981 and 1983, the incidence of tuberculosis fell by almost 15%. The decrease was less than 9% between 1983 and 1985 and less than 1%

between 1985 and 1987. Between 1987 and 1989, the incidence increased by more than 2%.

When the percentage change in reported cases of tuberculosis between 1985 and 1988 is examined by age, a striking pattern is apparent (Figure 3–10). For all age groups except 25–44 years, the number of reported cases fell during this time period. In contrast, the 25–44-year group experienced a substantial rise in reported disease. The percentage increase in the 25–44-year group was particularly high for Hispanics (35%) and blacks (23%). These patterns primarily reflect the emergence of clinically active tuberculosis among persons infected with HIV.

The usual rate of occurrence for a disease in a population is referred to as the **endemic rate.** A rapid and dramatic increase over the endemic rate is described as an **epidemic rate.** The development of an epidemic as a function of time is illustrated schematically in Figure 3–11. For an acute condition, such as a viral illness, the epidemic may develop over a matter of days or weeks. In contrast, for a chronic illness, such as lung cancer, the epidemic may emerge over a period of years to decades.

The time lag or **latent period** between exposure to a risk factor and diagnosis of a disease can be as short as a few hours (eg, staphylococcal food poisoning) to decades (eg, infection to clinically active tuberculosis). Obviously, the greater the time between the

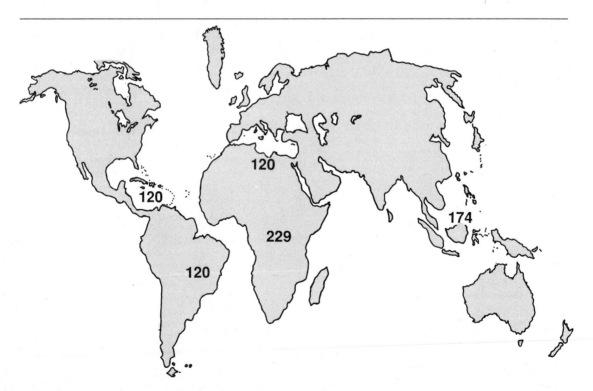

**Figure 3–6.** Estimated incidence rates per 100,000 person-years for tuberculosis in regions of the developing world in 1990. (Data from CDC: Tuberculosis in developing countries. MMWR 1990;39:561.)

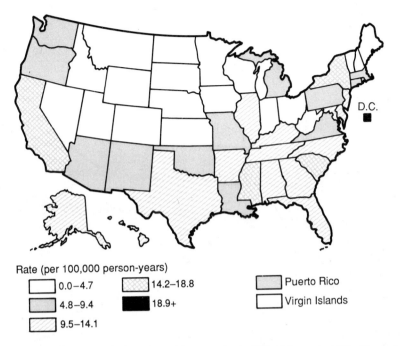

Rate (per 100,000 person-years)

0.0–4.7  14.2–18.8  Puerto Rico
4.8–9.4  18.9+  Virgin Islands
9.5–14.1

**Figure 3–7.** Incidence rates for tuberculosis, grouped by state, in the United States in 1989. (Reproduced from CDC: Summary of notifiable diseases, United States, 1989. MMWR 1990;38:1.)

occurrence of an initiating event and recognition of disease, the more difficult it may be to establish the linkage between risk factor and disease occurrence. This task is made even more challenging if the risk factor is a weak determinant of the disease or if multiple different risk factors are involved.

As noted earlier, the incidence of tuberculosis in the United States ended a long-term continuous decline in 1984. At the prior rate of decline, one would have expected almost 15,000 fewer cases to occur between 1984 and 1988 (Figure 3–12). This increase in disease occurrence does not represent an epidemic in the conventional sense of a rapid rise in incidence. It does indicate a departure from the prior downward

trend, however, and suggests that some new force began influencing tuberculosis incidence after 1984.

Several observations support the speculation that HIV influenced the observed trend in tuberculosis incidence:

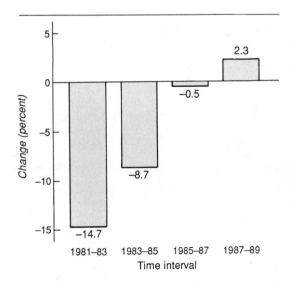

**Figure 3–9.** Percentage change in the incidence rate per 100,000 person-years for tuberculosis, grouped by 3-year time interval, in the United States, 1981–89. (Data from CDC: Summary of notifiable diseases, United States, 1989. MMWR 1990;38:1.)

**Figure 3–8.** Incidence rates for tuberculosis by year in the United States, 1980–89. (Data from CDC: Summary of notifiable diseases, United States, 1989. MMWR 1990; 38:1.)

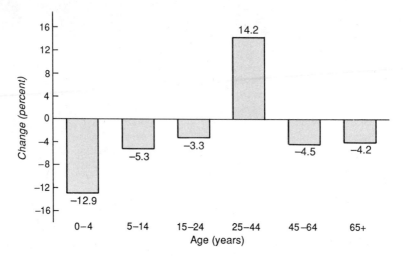

**Figure 3–10.** Percentage change in the number of reported cases of tuberculosis by age in the United States between 1985 and 1988. (Data from CDC: Update: Tuberculosis elimination–United States. MMWR 1990;39:153.)

**(1)** AIDS emerged at about the same time as the decline in tuberculosis ended.

**(2)** The age groups most affected by AIDS also have experienced an increase in tuberculosis incidence.

**(3)** The incidence of both AIDS and tuberculosis has increased considerably in black and Hispanic populations since 1984.

**(4)** The immune dysfunction associated with HIV infection facilitates progression from latent to clinically active tuberculosis.

**(5)** Clinical studies have revealed that a high proportion of persons infected with HIV have a history of tuberculosis, and conversely, a high proportion of tuberculosis patients in certain populations are seropositive for HIV.

The actual impact of HIV infection on the trends in tuberculosis morbidity is uncertain, because individual tuberculosis case report forms do not include information on HIV status. Nevertheless, it appears reasonable to conclude that the recent trend in the incidence of tuberculosis has been influenced substantially by HIV.

## CORRELATIONS WITH DISEASE OCCURRENCE

In order to develop hypotheses about possible causes of disease occurrence, the presence of a suspected risk factor can be measured in different populations and compared with the incidence of a particular disease. This type of comparison is referred to as an **ecologic study,** because the analysis is at the level of an entire population, rather than at the level of individual persons. Another name for this type of investigation is **correlation study,** since it seeks to determine the extent to which two characteristics (risk factor and disease occurrence) are related.

An example of ecologic data is shown in Figure 3–13. In this graph, the incidence rates of AIDS in 13 states of the United States during 1989 are compared with corresponding incidence rates of tuberculosis for that same year. The states included in this analysis (New York, Pennsylvania, Massachusetts, Florida, Georgia, Kentucky, Texas, Illinois, Kansas, Iowa, Utah, California, and Washington) were selected because they represented diverse geographic areas with varying demographic characteristics.

In general, the states that had a high incidence of AIDS also had a high incidence of tuberculosis (eg, New York, Florida, California). At the other extreme, states with a low incidence of AIDS also tended to have a low incidence of tuberculosis (eg, Iowa, Utah, Kansas). As a general rule, the incidence of AIDS

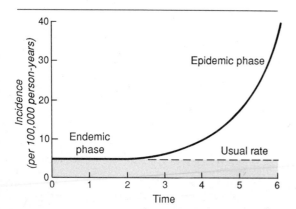

**Figure 3–11.** Schematic representation of the development of an epidemic of disease over time.

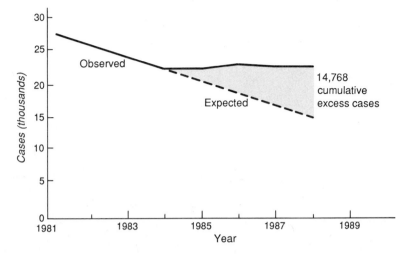

**Figure 3–12.** Observed and expected numbers of tuberculosis cases in the United States, 1981–88. (Reproduced from CDC: Tuberculosis elimination–United States. MMWR 1990;39:153.)

was about twice the corresponding incidence of tuberculosis. A few exceptions occurred, such as Kentucky, where the incidence of AIDS (3.0 cases per 100,000 person-years) was considerably less than the incidence of tuberculosis (10.2 cases per 100,000 person-years).

In order to assess the strength of the relationship between AIDS and tuberculosis incidence, a correlation analysis was performed (see *Basic and Clinical Biostatistics* [Dawson-Saunders and Trapp, 1990]). The correlation coefficient was 0.86, which indicated that the incidence of AIDS and tuberculosis were strongly and positively related. The **coefficient of determination,** the square of the correlation coefficient, was 0.75. This means that 75% of the vari-

ability in the incidence of tuberculosis could be accounted for by knowing the AIDS incidence.

A linear regression analysis of these data (see Dawson-Saunders and Trapp, 1990) yielded the following equation:

$$\text{Tuberculosis IR} = 3.25 + 0.44 \times (\text{AIDS IR})$$

The graph of this regression line is depicted in Figure 3–14. In this analysis, the effect of AIDS incidence in determining the incidence of tuberculosis is highly statistically significant. In other words, it is very unlikely that the observed relationship between AIDS and tuberculosis incidence rates occurred by chance

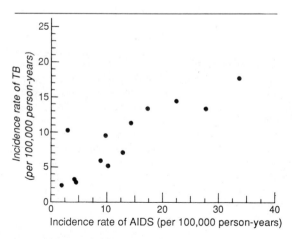

**Figure 3–13.** Scatterplot of the incidence rates of AIDS and tuberculosis (TB) in thirteen states of the United States, 1989. (Data from CDC: Summary of notifiable diseases, United States, 1989. MMWR 1990;38:1.)

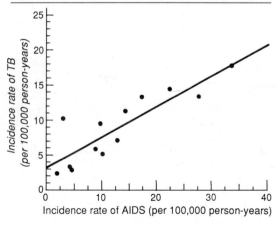

**Figure 3–14.** Regression line for regression of tuberculosis (TB) incidence on AIDS incidence in thirteen states of the United States, 1989. (Data from CDC: Summary of notifiable diseases, United States, 1989. MMWR 1990; 38:1.)

alone. From the regression equation it also can be seen that in the absence of AIDS (AIDS incidence = 0 cases per 100,000 person-years), the expected incidence of tuberculosis is 3.25 cases per 100,000 person-years. For every increase of one case per 100,000 person-years in the AIDS incidence, the tuberculosis incidence is expected to increase by 0.44 cases per 100,000 person-years.

The relationship depicted in Figure 3–14 is very striking and suggests that the occurrence of AIDS may influence the development of tuberculosis. This type of correlation analysis, however, is best viewed as a **hypothesis-generating** study, which means that it can help formulate a hypothesis about the link between these two diseases but it cannot establish a causal relationship between them. A correlation between AIDS and tuberculosis incidence could occur for reasons other than a cause-and-effect relationship. For example, risk factors for both diseases (eg, intravenous drug use) might be the true reason for the apparent association between AIDS and tuberculosis.

Studies that are designed to test the likelihood of a cause-and-effect relationship between a risk factor and a disease are termed **hypothesis-testing** investigations. The two approaches most commonly employed to test associations between risk factors and disease are cohort and case-control studies. These research designs are described in Chapters 8 and 9, respectively. The effects of related variables, such as intravenous drug use, can be considered in the design and analysis of these studies.

An important limitation on the epidemiologist's ability to infer a causal explanation from a correlation study is the **ecologic fallacy.** This problem may occur when a suspected risk factor and disease occurrence are associated at the population level, but not at the individual subject level. In other words, populations may have high incidence rates of AIDS (risk factor) and of tuberculosis (disease occurrence) without the same persons being affected by both conditions. This type of ecologic fallacy can be avoided only by making observations of risk factor and disease status on individual subjects. Methods of analytic epidemiology, such as cohort and case-control studies, involve observations on individuals, and thus are not subject to the hazards of ecologic reasoning.

## MIGRATION AND DISEASE OCCURRENCE

Another useful technique in descriptive epidemiology is the examination of the effects of migration on the rate of disease occurrence. Studies of this type can help clarify whether a disease of unknown cause is determined principally by genetic inheritance or by environmental exposure. As depicted in Figure 3–15, migration from a high-risk population to a low-risk population should not affect the occurrence of a genetically determined disease among the migrants. In

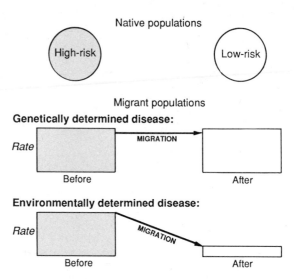

**Figure 3–15.** Schematic representation of the effects of migration on the rates of occurrence of genetically and environmentally determined diseases.

contrast, migration from a high-risk population to a low-risk population is expected to be associated with a reduction in occurrence of an environmentally determined disease. Expressed in another way, migration diminishes the likelihood of exposure to environmental risk factors, and accordingly, the occurrence of disease should decrease. Of course, for diseases with long latent periods, it may take many years for the reduced rate of occurrence to become manifest. If environmental exposures early in life are critical, then the rate of occurrence may not be reduced among the migrants themselves (who were exposed prior to their departure), but should be diminished among their offspring born in the new location. A dramatic change in disease incidence within a single generation could not be explained on the basis of genetic changes.

A number of studies have indicated that a progressive decline over time in the incidence of tuberculosis occurs among persons who migrate from high-risk areas (eg, Asia) to low-risk areas (eg, the United States, western Europe). The basic pattern of change in incidence is shown in Figure 3–16. The incidence of tuberculosis is highest at the time of migration and falls rapidly in the next few years. The decline continues, with smaller increments of change over time, for many years. The incidence among migrants does not fall to the level of the general population, however, presumably because of latent infections acquired prior to migration. Other factors that may contribute to the persistence of elevated incidence of tuberculosis among migrants include:

• Residence in migrant communities, thus maintaining a comparatively high rate of disease transmission

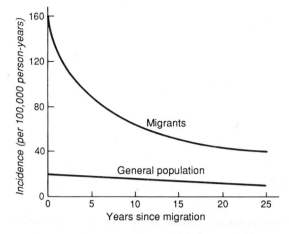

**Figure 3–16.** Comparison of the incidence of tuberculosis among migrants who moved from high- to low-risk countries with the incidence in the general population of the adopted country.

- Crowded housing conditions
- Poor nutritional status
- Inadequate access to preventive or therapeutic medical services
- Noncompliance with therapy
- Presence of tuberculosis that is resistant to conventional antibiotics
- Reinfection upon return visits to the country of origin

The overall decline in incidence of tuberculosis among migrants from high- to low-risk countries, however, provides strong circumstantial evidence about the importance of environmental determinants of this disease.

## SUMMARY

In this chapter, the basic approaches to descriptive epidemiology were presented, with a focus on the patterns of occurrence of tuberculosis. Description in epidemiology begins with the assumption that diseases do not occur at random. Three standard questions typically are posed to characterize the nonrandom distribution of a disease: (1) **Who** gets the disease? (2) **Where** does the disease occur? and (3) **When** does the disease occur? These questions concern the elements of **person, place,** and **time,** respectively.

At a minimum, the personal attributes examined in relation to disease occurrence are the distributions by age, race, and sex. The incidence of tuberculosis in the United States increases with advancing age. The racial/ethnic groups with the highest occurrence of this disease are Asians and Pacific Islanders, blacks, Hispanics, and Native Americans and Alaskan Natives. In addition, males have higher incidence rates for tuberculosis than do females.

The place of occurrence of a disease may be studied at the international, regional, or local level. Tuberculosis occurs with great excess in the nonindustrialized countries. Even within an industrialized country, such as the United States, substantial regional and local variation in incidence is reported.

Temporal patterns can be examined across years, months, or days, depending upon the time course of the disease in question. For tuberculosis, a progressive decline in incidence over time was observed in the United States until 1984, with minimal change thereafter. The change in the temporal pattern of this disease, suggested that the introduction of a new factor around 1984, probably HIV, altered the occurrence of tuberculosis.

The concept of an **epidemic** as a rapid and dramatic increase in the incidence of a disease was introduced with analogy to the greater than expected occurrence of tuberculosis after 1984. The use of **ecologic** (or correlation) **studies** was illustrated by a comparison of incidence rates of AIDS and tuberculosis in selected states. In an ecologic study, the overall amount of a risk factor (eg, AIDS) is related to the occurrence of a disease (eg, tuberculosis) across different populations. This type of correlation can be useful for **generating hypotheses,** but not for testing causal relationships. The influence of a background variable that is related both to the presumed causal factor and the outcome of interest can limit the utility of a correlation analysis. Furthermore, the **ecologic fallacy** can lead to a misleading conclusion when the risk factor and disease are related at the population level but not within particular individuals.

Finally, the use of studies of disease occurrence in relation to migration patterns in order to distinguish genetic from environmental origins was discussed. As applied to tuberculosis, persons who migrate from high-risk areas (eg, Asia) to low-risk areas (eg, the United States and western Europe) experience a progressive decline in incidence over time. This pattern strongly indicates that the primary influences on the occurrence of tuberculosis are environmental.

## STUDY QUESTIONS

**Directions:** For each question, select the single best answer.

1. Data on the number of cases of shigellosis reported among persons aged 25 years or older in the United States for 1989 are shown by age in Table 3–3. It cannot be concluded from this information that the 30–39-year age group is at the highest risk among the age groups shown because:
   A. The ecologic fallacy may be present
   B. The data are for one year only
   C. The sizes of the source populations by age are not given

**Table 3–3.** Number of shigellosis cases reported, by age, among persons 25 years or older in the United States for 1989.[1]

| Age | Number of Cases |
|---|---|
| 25–29 | 1457 |
| 30–39 | 1929 |
| 40–49 | 846 |
| 50–59 | 451 |
| 60+ | 640 |

[1]Data from CDC: Summary of notifiable diseases, United States, 1989. MMWR 1990;38:1.

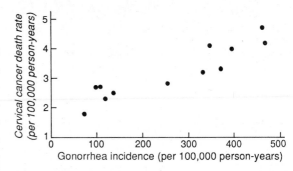

**Figure 3–17.** Scatterplot of the incidence of gonorrhea in 1989 and age-adjusted death rate from cervical cancer in 1984–88 in selected states of the United States. (Data on gonorrhea from CDC: Summary of notifiable diseases, United States, 1989. MMWR 1990;38:1. Data on cervical cancer from Ries LAG et al: *Cancer Statistics Review, 1973–88.* NIH Publication No. 91–2789. National Cancer Institute, 1991.)

    D. The places of occurrence are not known
    E. No comparison group is included

2. Likely explanations for the high incidence rates of tuberculosis among Hispanics compared to non-Hispanic whites in the United States include each of the following EXCEPT
    A. Migration from areas with high incidence
    B. Crowded living conditions
    C. Inadequate access to preventive health services
    D. Poor nutritional status
    E. The relatively small size of the source population

3. The country with the highest incidence of tuberculosis among the following is:
    A. Italy
    B. Philippines
    C. Spain
    D. Canada
    E. United States

4. Which of the following reasons is LEAST likely to explain the declining incidence of reported cases of clinically active tuberculosis in the United States between 1940 and 1984?
    A. Chlorination of drinking water supplies
    B. Better housing conditions
    C. Antibiotic therapy
    D. Improved nutritional status

5. The latent period is defined as the time from:
    A. Birth until first exposure to a risk factor
    B. Initial to final exposure to a risk factor
    C. Exposure to a risk factor until occurrence of the disease
    D. Disease occurrence until death
    E. First until last case occurrence

6. The usual incidence of a disease in a population is referred to as the:
    A. Pandemic rate
    B. Epidemic rate
    C. Hypodermic rate
    D. Endemic rate
    E. Hyperdemic rate

**Questions 7–9:** Figure 3–17 is a scatterplot of the incidence of gonorrhea and the death rate from cervical cancer in Alabama, California, Colorado, Illinois, Iowa, Louisiana, Massachusetts, Minnesota, New York, Oregon, South Carolina, and Tennessee.

7. This type of study is best described as:
    A. Case-control
    B. Ecologic
    C. Cohort
    D. Randomized controlled trial
    E. Case series

8. The correlation coefficient for these data is closest to:
    A. −0.9
    B. −0.1
    C. 0
    D. +0.1
    E. +0.9

9. This analysis does not establish a cause-and-effect relationship between gonorrhea and cervical cancer because:
    A. Only 12 states were studied
    B. Insufficient variation in cervical cancer mortality was observed
    C. There is no comparison group
    D. Another factor related to gonorrhea could be the true cause of cervical cancer
    E. Not all cases of gonorrhea were reported

10. Which of the following diseases is LEAST likely to change in incidence for the offspring of migrants who leave a high-risk country and move to a low-risk country?
    A. Cystic fibrosis
    B. Stroke
    C. Malaria
    D. Unintentional injury
    E. Coronary artery disease

## FURTHER READING

Rieder HL: Epidemiology of tuberculosis in the United States. Epidemiol Rev 1989;11:79.

## REFERENCES

### Clinical Background

CDC: Screening for tuberculosis infection in high-risk populations and the use of preventive therapy for tuberculosis infection in the United States. MMWR 1990;39(RR-8):1.

CDC: Guidelines for preventing the transmission of tuberculosis in health care settings, with special focus on HIV-related issues. MMWR 1990;39(RR-17):1.

### Descriptive Epidemiology

CDC: Summary of notifiable diseases, United States, 1989. MMWR 1990;38:1.

CDC: Update: Tuberculosis elimination–United States. MMWR 1990;39:153.

CDC: Tuberculosis in developing countries. MMWR 1990;39:561.

### Epidemic Disease Occurrence

CDC: Tuberculosis and human immunodeficiency virus infection: Recommendations of the Advisory Committee for the Elimination of Tuberculosis (ACET). MMWR 1989;38:236.

### Correlations with Disease Occurrence

CDC: Summary of notifiable diseases, United States, 1989. MMWR 1990;38:1.

Dawson-Saunders B, Trapp RG: *Basic and Clinical Biostatistics.* Appleton & Lange, 1990.

### Migration and Disease Occurrence

Medical Research Council Tuberculosis and Chest Diseases Unit: National survey of notifications of tuberculosis in England and Wales in 1983. BMJ 1985;291:658.

# Medical Surveillance

## PATIENT PROFILE

*A 68-year-old female retired office manager presented with a dry, hacking cough of several months' duration. She reported a history of smoking one pack of cigarettes per day for the past 30 years. In order to evaluate the patient's cough, her family physician ordered a chest x-ray, which was unremarkable except for an increased density in the hilum (midcentral portion) of the lung fields. A sputum specimen was collected and abnormally appearing cells were noted upon microscopic evaluation. Since these cells might be cancerous, a bronchoscopic examination was performed to allow direct visualization of the large airways. A partially obstructing mass was visible at the distal end of the right main stem bronchus. Brushings from this mass revealed cells consistent with a diagnosis of squamous cell carcinoma. Other diagnostic studies indicated that the cancer had spread to involve the brain and bones. Radiation therapy was administered to all sites of cancer involvement. Nevertheless, the patient's condition rapidly deteriorated and she died less than 6 months after diagnosis.*

## INTRODUCTION

In this chapter, attention is focused on one of the most basic functions of epidemiology: *detection of the occurrence of health-related events or exposures in a target population.* The goal of this detection, or **surveillance,** is to identify changes in the distributions of diseases in order to prevent or control these diseases within a population. The term surveillance literally means "to watch over," and traditionally medical surveillance activities were developed to monitor the spread of infectious diseases through a population. Today, however, surveillance programs have been applied to a wide variety of other conditions, such as congenital malformations, injuries, occupational health problems, and cancer, as well as other behaviors that affect health. Regardless of the type of outcome under consideration, medical surveillance activities involve the following key features:

- Continuous data collection and evaluation
- An identified target population (such as a community, a work force, or a group of patients)

- A standard definition of the outcome of interest
- Emphasis upon timeliness of collection and dissemination of information
- Use of data for purposes of investigation or disease control

The goals of a medical surveillance activity depend upon the state of knowledge about the causes of the condition of interest and the extent to which effective preventive measures are known (Table 4–1). Surveillance activities can provide data about the distribution of a disease by person, place, and time. These patterns of occurrence can help to shed light on possible causes of the disease. For example, if the time and place of disease occurrence are similar for two or more subjects, a shared source of illness, such as an infectious agent, may be involved. Other demographic information about affected individuals, such as age, race, and gender, typically are collected during surveillance and may provide further insight into the modes of disease acquisition. More detailed information on the personal characteristics of affected individuals can be collected through personal interviews.

In the following sections, various aspects of medical surveillance will be described. By relating each of these activities to the diagnosis of lung cancer in the Patient Profile, an attempt will be made to demonstrate the interrelationships between different types of surveillance.

## SURVEILLANCE OF NEW DIAGNOSES

In the United States, the incidence of cancer is monitored by the National Cancer Institute through a network of population-based registries, collectively comprising the Surveillance, Epidemiology, and End Results (SEER) program. The expression **population-based** means that the target group is the general population delimited by place of residence, and the term is used to contrast with other registries, such as hospital-based or industry-based surveys.

At present, there are nine areas involved in the SEER program, which incorporate entire states (Utah, Iowa, Connecticut, New Mexico, and Hawaii) as well as metropolitan regions (Atlanta, Detroit,

**Table 4–1.** Possible goals of medical surveillance activities.

Identification of patterns of disease occurrence
Detection of disease outbreaks
Development of clues about possible risk factors
Finding of cases for further investigation
Anticipation of health service needs

Seattle, and San Francisco) (Figure 4–1). Although almost 10% of the population of the United States resides within these nine areas combined, this is clearly not a random sample of the nation. The areas were selected largely on the basis of ability to maintain ongoing population-based cancer reporting systems and epidemiologic interest in the population subgroups that reside there. Collectively these registries provide reasonably representative samples of different regions of the country, rural and urban populations, and most major racial and ethnic groups.

The SEER registries use a variety of methods to locate new diagnoses of cancer. The vast majority of diagnoses are identified from hospital admissions through the review of pathology reports and lists of discharge diagnoses. Additional sources of cases include pathology laboratories outside of hospitals, office records of physicians, outpatient treatment facilities, and death certificates. The size of the population at risk of cancer is derived for each geographic area by extrapolation from census estimates.

The 1988 annual age-adjusted incidence rates for the five most common types of cancer among men and women of all races in the United States are shown in Figure 4–2. By convention the incidence rates for cancer are expressed per 100,000 person-years. The

incidence rate for lung cancer means that 58 individuals within a representative sample of 100,000 persons in the United States are expected to develop lung cancer in one year.

The incidence of lung cancer is twice as high among males as among females in the United States. Moreover, as illustrated in Figure 4–3, the incidence of lung cancer is not constant across age groups. This disease is extremely rare in persons under 40 years of age. After age 40 the incidence of lung cancer rises sharply, reaching a plateau among persons in their 70s.

The striking relationship between age and incidence of lung cancer (and most other types of cancer as well) creates a potential complication in comparing the incidence rates of population groups of differing age distributions. In other words, simply because of their relative youth, a younger group of individuals will tend to have fewer occurrences of lung cancer than an older group of people. Failure to account for this age discrepancy would result in a distorted comparison of lung cancer incidence rates between the two groups. In order to allow a comparison of incidence rates that is not influenced by age differences in the underlying populations, one must perform an age-adjustment procedure. The usual approach is, referred to as **direct age adjustment** (or direct age standardization), in which *a single standard age structure is applied to the age-specific incidence rates for the groups being compared, resulting in summary rates for the groups that are not distorted by differences in age.* For direct age adjustment of cancer incidence rates in the United States, the standard age distribution used is that of the entire population of the

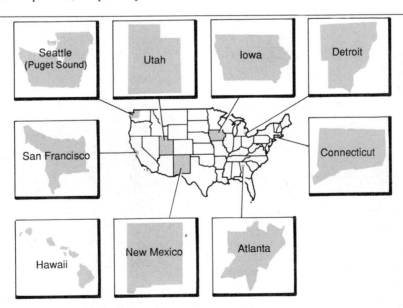

**Figure 4–1.** Geographic distribution of data collection centers involved in the SEER program. (Modified and reproduced from Ries LAG et al: *Cancer Statistics Review, 1973–88.* National Cancer Institute. NIH Publication No. 91–2789, 1991.)

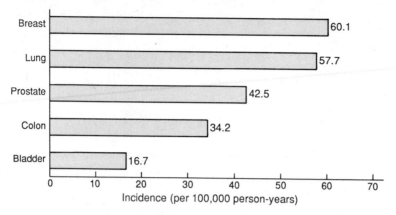

**Figure 4–2.** Incidence rates for the five leading forms of cancer in the United States, 1988. (Data from Ries LAG et al: *Cancer Statistics Review, 1973–88.* National Cancer Institute. NIH Publication No. 91–2789, 1991.)

country in 1970. Summary lung cancer incidence rates for whites and blacks, for example, can be compared for any calendar year by determining the rate of cancer that would have occurred in each racial group if they had the age distribution of the US population in 1970. The choice of the standard age distribution is arbitrary—any distribution can be used as long as it is applied equally to the groups under comparison. The topic of age adjustment is presented in greater detail later in this chapter and in *Basic and Clinical Biostatistics* (Dawson-Saunders and Trapp, 1990).

## RATE COMPARISONS

The age-adjusted incidence rates for leading forms of cancer in the United States are shown by race in Table 4–2. From these data, it can be seen that if the

effect of age is held constant, blacks tend to have higher rates of occurrence of lung cancer and prostate cancer than do whites. In contrast, bladder cancer tends to occur with greater incidence among whites than blacks. For breast and colon cancers, rates of occurrence do not differ greatly between the races, although there is a slightly higher incidence of breast cancer among whites and a small elevation of colon cancer occurrence among blacks.

By dividing the incidence rate among blacks by the incidence rate among whites, a summary measure of disparity in rates of occurrence is obtained. An index of the racial disparity in cancer incidence is the ratio of black-to-white incidence rates, or **rate ratio** (RR). If blacks and whites have the same rate of disease occurrence, the rate ratio would have a value of unity (RR = 1). When blacks have an elevated incidence compared to whites, the black-to-white rate ratio is greater than one (RR > 1). In contrast, when blacks have a lower occurrence rate than do whites, the rate ratio is less than one (RR < 1). The further the RR is

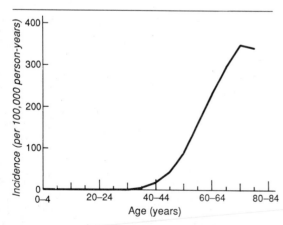

**Figure 4–3.** Age-specific incidence rates for lung cancer in the United States, 1984–88. (Data from Ries LAG et al: *Cancer Statistics Review, 1973–88.* National Cancer Institute. NIH Publication No. 91–2789, 1991.)

**Table 4–2.** The annual age-adjusted incidence rates per 100,000 person-years in whites and blacks for leading forms of cancer in the United States in 1988.[1]

| Type of Cancer | Incidence Rate[4] | | Black-to-White Rate Ratio |
| --- | --- | --- | --- |
| | Blacks | Whites | |
| Breast[2] | 96.5 | 112.9 | 0.9 |
| Lung | 74.4 | 57.7 | 1.3 |
| Prostate[3] | 136.0 | 101.9 | 1.3 |
| Colon | 38.1 | 33.8 | 1.1 |
| Bladder | 8.5 | 18.0 | 0.5 |

[1] Data from Ries LAG et al: *Cancer Statistics Review, 1973–88.* National Cancer Institute. NIH Publication No. 91–2789, 1991.
[2] Females only.
[3] Males only.
[4] Directly age adjusted to the 1970 population of the USA.

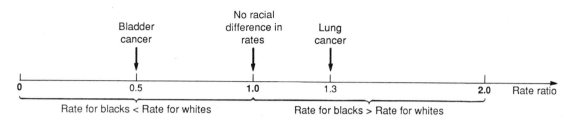

**Figure 4–4.** Schematic representation of black-to-white incidence rate ratio for cancers of the lung and bladder in the United States.

away from unity, the greater the disparity in incidence between the races.

The black-to-white rate ratio of 1.3 for lung cancer indicates that the incidence of this cancer in black persons is about one-third greater than it is in whites (Figure 4–4). In contrast, the rate ratio of 0.5 for bladder cancer indicates that the incidence of this cancer in blacks is about one-half as high as that in whites. These patterns suggest that the factors that influence the development of lung cancer and the factors that influence the development of bladder cancer are distributed differently between the races. These predisposing conditions, termed **risk factors,** could include genetic susceptibility to the cancers in question, as well as exposure to environmental agents.

Variation in incidence across demographic groups can provide important leads about the causation of specific types of cancers. For example, cigarette smoking has been linked to the development of both lung and bladder cancers, and a larger proportion of blacks than whites smoke. Thus, racial differences in cigarette smoking may account for the increased occurrence of lung cancer among blacks. The higher incidence of bladder cancer among whites, however, suggests that factors in addition to cigarette smoking must be involved in the development of this disease.

## SURVEILLANCE OF DEATHS

Another index used to measure the population distribution of a disease is the **mortality rate,** which characterizes the rapidity with which deaths from the disease occur over time. The mortality rate is determined by the combined forces of the rate of new diagnoses **(incidence rate),** and the likelihood of death following diagnosis **(case fatality).** For diseases with a high case fatality (a low rate of cure or recovery), such as lung cancer, mortality rates give a reasonable approximation of incidence rates. As shown in Figure 4–5, the overall age-adjusted mortality rate for lung cancer is about three-fourths as great as the corresponding incidence rate. A malignancy with a more favorable prognosis, such as thyroid cancer, will have a greater disparity between mortality and incidence rates (Figure 4–6). The age-adjusted mor-

tality rate for thyroid cancer is only about one-tenth as large as the corresponding incidence rate, since most persons who develop this disease do not die from it.

Despite the potential disparity between incidence and mortality rates, the distribution of deaths from a disease by person, place, and time still can be useful for surveillance purposes. Pragmatic advantages to the use of mortality information for surveillance purposes are listed below.

* Widely collected, virtually complete data (registration of deaths is compulsory in most industrialized countries, and few deaths are not reported)
* Standardized nomenclature (the International Classification of Diseases is used to promote uniformity in reporting of causes of death)
* Modest cost (recording of deaths is relatively inexpensive)

Mortality statistics thus serve as a convenient tool for epidemiologic surveillance, particularly when incidence data are not available. For example, as already noted, the SEER program covers less than 10% of the population of the United States, but death registration is compulsory throughout the nation. Accordingly, mortality statistics can provide a more complete picture of the geographic distribution of cancer than can be determined from incidence data alone. A map of age-adjusted mortality rates for lung cancer

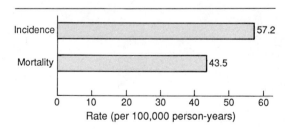

**Figure 4–5.** Age-adjusted incidence and mortality rates for lung cancer in the United States, 1984–88. (Data from Ries LAG et al: *Cancer Statistics Review, 1973–88.* National Cancer Institute. NIH Publication No. 91–2789, 1991.)

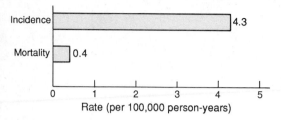

**Figure 4–6.** Age-adjusted incidence and mortality rates for thyroid cancer in the United States, 1984–88. (Data from Ries LAG et al: *Cancer Statistics Review, 1973–88.* National Cancer Institute. NIH Publication No. 91–2789, 1991.)

for whites in the United States illustrates this point (Figure 4–7).

As shown in Figure 4–8, the process of collecting information on deaths in the United States begins with completion of a death certificate by an attending physician, medical examiner, or coroner. The conditions responsible, in whole or in part, for the patient's death are recorded on the certificate. Standard coding rules are utilized to determine the underlying **cause of death,** which is defined as (1) the disease or injury which initiated the train of morbid events leading directly to death, or (2) the circumstances of the accident or violence that resulted in the fatal injury. Death certificates are aggregated at the state level by vital statistics offices. The information is then transferred

to the National Center for Health Statistics for compilation into a nationwide data base.

## AGE ADJUSTMENT

Mortality rates for all causes of death in the United States are shown by age and race in Figure 4–9. For both whites and blacks, mortality rates begin at high levels during the first year of life, fall to low levels during childhood, adolescence, and young adulthood, and then rise rapidly with increasing age. At every age, however, the death rates for blacks exceed those of whites.

It might be surprising, therefore, that the **crude death rate** (total deaths/total person-years) for blacks (874 deaths/100,000 person-years) is comparable to the corresponding rate for whites (905 deaths/100,000 person-years). As indicated in Figure 4–10, the black-to-white ratio of mortality rates is 0.97, indicating virtually no difference between the races in the rate of deaths. This apparent paradox is explained by differences in the underlying age distributions of blacks and whites. On average, black persons in the United States tend to be younger than whites (Figure 4–11). For example, only 8.4% of blacks in the United States are 65 years or older, compared to 13.2% of whites. Thus, a smaller proportion of the black population experiences the high mortality associated with advanced age. In order to obtain an un-

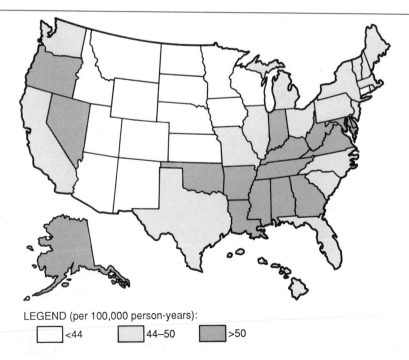

LEGEND (per 100,000 person-years): ☐ <44  ☐ 44–50  ■ >50

**Figure 4–7.** The age-adjusted lung cancer mortality rates for whites by state, United States, 1984–88. (Reproduced from Ries LAG et al: *Cancer Statistics Review, 1973–88.* National Cancer Institute. NIH Publication No. 91–2789, 1991.)

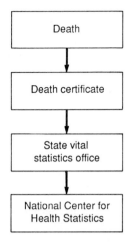

**Figure 4–8.** Flow diagram for processing of information about deaths in the United States.

distorted summary comparison of mortality for blacks and whites, the age differential between the races must be estimated.

As noted previously, the usual approach to removing the influence of age from a comparison of summary rates is direct age adjustment. This technique involves the following steps:

(1) Select a standard age structure. By convention, the standard distribution used for age adjustment of mortality rates in the United States is the age distribution of the total population of the country in 1940.
(2) Multiply the age-specific mortality rates for each group being compared by the corresponding age-specific numbers of persons in the standard popu-

lation. The result is the expected number of deaths for that age group.
(3) Sum the expected numbers of deaths within each age group to yield a total number of expected deaths for each group being compared.
(4) Divide the total number of expected deaths in each group by the total size of the standard population to yield the summary age-adjusted mortality rate.

When this direct age-adjustment procedure is performed on the age-specific death rates for blacks and whites in the United States for 1988, the summary mortality rates shown in Figure 4–12 are obtained. Note that the age-adjusted rates are lower than the corresponding crude rates (Figure 4–10) for both racial groups. Since the 1940 standard population tended to be skewed toward younger ages than either the black or white populations of 1988, the age-adjusted rates are lower than the crude rates. The change for whites is greater than that for blacks because of a larger differential between the standard (1940) and the more recent (1988) age distribution.

The numerical values of the age-adjusted rates are not particularly meaningful by themselves, since the values will vary according to the standard age distribution used. The utility of the age-adjusted rates is that they allow comparisons across groups, such as the black-to-white rate ratio. It can be seen from Figure 4–12 that the age-adjusted mortality rate for blacks is more than 50% larger than it is for whites (rate ratio = 1.55). Thus, the age-adjusted mortality rate ratio provides a summary measure that is consistent with the increase in black mortality shown in Figure 4–9. Through the use of an adjustment technique, the distorting effect of age has been removed from the contrast of summary mortality rates.

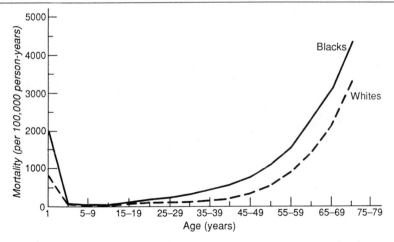

**Figure 4–9.** Mortality rates for all causes of death in the United States, by age and race, 1988. (Data from National Center for Health Statistics: Advance report of final mortality statistics, 1988. Monthly Vital Statistics Report. Vol 39, No. 7 [Suppl], 1990.)

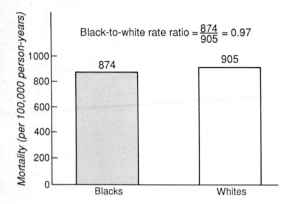

$$\text{Black-to-white rate ratio} = \frac{874}{905} = 0.97$$

**Figure 4–10.** Crude mortality rates for blacks and whites in the United States, 1988. (Data from National Center for Health Statistics: Advance report of final mortality statistics, 1988. Monthly Vital Statistics Report. Vol 39, No. 7 [Suppl], 1990.)

## MORTALITY PATTERNS

In addition to variation by age and race, mortality in the United Sates also varies by other characteristics. Age-adjusted mortality rates for whites and blacks for calendar years 1978 through 1988 are shown in Figure 4–13. Among whites, mortality has continued to decline through this entire time period. For blacks, progressive decreases in mortality were observed through 1984, with slight increases thereafter.

As shown in Figure 4–14, black males have the highest age-adjusted mortality rate, followed in succession by white males and black females, with the lowest death rates observed among white females. Within both racial groups, males have higher mortality rates than do females. For both genders, blacks have higher mortality rates than do whites.

The annual age-adjusted mortality rates for all persons combined in the United States are listed for the ten leading causes of death in Table 4–3. Four of the five most common causes of death in this country result from long-term, chronic processes: heart diseases, malignant neoplasms (cancer), cerebrovascular diseases (stroke), and chronic obstructive pulmonary diseases.

Mortality rates for the individual causes of death vary by race and gender. Blacks have higher death rates than whites for eight of the ten leading causes of death (Figure 4–15). The relative increase in mortality among blacks is greatest for nephritis, nephrotic syndrome, and nephrosis (black-to-white rate ratio = 2.8), followed by diabetes mellitus (RR = 2.4), stroke (RR = 1.9), and chronic liver disease/cirrhosis (RR = 1.7). Only suicide (RR = 0.6) and chronic obstructive pulmonary diseases (RR = 0.8) are responsible for lower rates of death among blacks than whites.

As depicted in Figure 4–16, males have higher mortality rates for all of the ten leading causes of death in the United States. The relative increase in mortality among males is greatest for suicide (male-to-female rate ratio = 4.0), unintentional injuries (RR = 2.7), chronic liver disease/cirrhosis (RR = 2.3), chronic obstructive pulmonary diseases (RR = 2.0), and heart diseases (RR = 1.9). The ratio of male-to-female death rates is lowest for diabetes mellitus (RR = 1.1) and stroke (RR = 1.2).

Trends in age-adjusted mortality rates for the ten

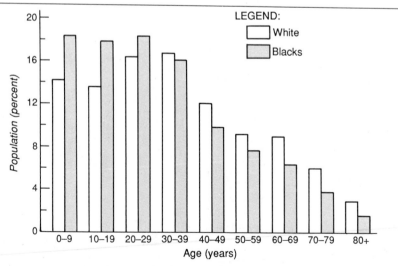

**Figure 4–11.** Age distributions of black and white persons in the United States, 1988. (Data determined from National Center for Health Statistics: Advance report of final mortality statistics, 1988. Monthly Vital Statistics Report. Vol 39, No. 7 [Suppl], 1990.)

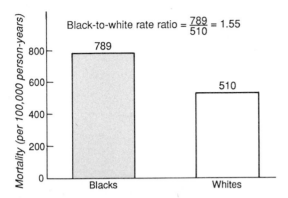

**Figure 4–12.** Age-adjusted (1940 US population standard) total mortality rates for blacks and whites in the United States, 1988. (Data from National Center for Health Statistics: Advance report of final mortality statistics, 1988. Monthly Vital Statistics Report. Vol 39, No. 7 [Suppl], 1990.)

leading causes of death over the time period 1979 through 1988 are displayed schematically in Figure 4–17. Dramatic declines in death rates occurred for stroke (−29%), chronic liver disease and cirrhosis (−25%), unintentional injuries (−18%), and heart diseases (−17%). Concurrent substantial percentage increases in mortality were seen for chronic obstructive pulmonary disease (+33%), pneumonia and influenza (+27%), and nephritis, nephrotic syndrome, and nephrosis (+12%).

Returning to lung cancer, the focus of the Patient Profile, the age-adjusted mortality rate from this disease is the highest for any form of cancer in the United States (Figure 4–18). Lung cancer accounts for more than one-fourth of all deaths from malignant neoplasms in the USA and more than twice the num-

ber of deaths as the next most common cause of death from cancer, malignancies of the large intestines. Between 1978 and 1988 (Figure 4–19) the age-adjusted mortality from lung cancer increased steadily in the United States. Overall, the rate of deaths from this disease increased by about 20% during this time period. As shown in Figure 4–20, the age-adjusted mortality from lung cancer varies considerably by race and gender in the United States. Among both whites and blacks, there is a considerably greater mortality from this disease among males. Black males have a more than 30% higher lung cancer death rate than white males. In contrast, virtually no racial differential in lung cancer mortality is seen among females.

## SURVEILLANCE OF RISK FACTORS

In the preceding section, attention was focused on surveillance of medical events, such as new diagnoses or deaths from specific diseases. Surveillance techniques also can be used to characterize patterns of risk factor distribution by person, place, and time. The Behavioral Risk Factor Surveillance System (BRFSS), which is supported by the Centers for Disease Control, collects this type of information. The BRFSS was initiated in 1984 in order to provide statewide data on lifestyle characteristics that could affect health status. Data are collected by the health departments of most states using a standard protocol. Adult respondents are sampled randomly and briefly interviewed over the telephone.

The most important risk factor for the development of lung cancer is cigarette smoking. Data collected by the BRFSS can be used to describe smoking patterns within the general population. The overall prevalence of cigarette smoking in the United States in 1988, as determined by the BRFSS, was 25%. As shown in Figure 4–21, the estimated prevalence of cigarette use varied by state of residence, with the highest reported level in Kentucky (34%) and the lowest reported level in Utah (15%). The low frequency of cigarette smoking in Utah is attributable to the high proportion of residents who practice Mormonism, a religion that advocates abstinence from tobacco and alcohol. Given the marked differential in cigarette smoking in Utah and Kentucky, it is not surprising that the age-adjusted lung cancer mortality in Utah is only about one-third as high as that in Kentucky.

Another system used to collect information on risk factors and health status in the United States is the National Health Interview Survey (NHIS). The NHIS is a continuous nationwide household survey, using data collected through personal interviews. In 1988 more than 120,000 persons were surveyed by the NHIS. The overall prevalence of current cigarette smoking in the United States during that year, as determined by the NHIS, was 28%. The slight difference in smoking prevalence estimates obtained by the

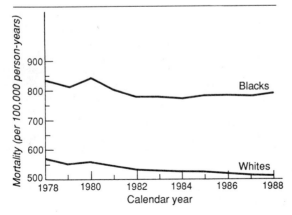

**Figure 4–13.** Age-adjusted total mortality rates by calendar year and race in the United States, 1978–88. (Data from National Center for Health Statistics: Advance report of final mortality statistics, 1988. Monthly Vital Statistics Report. Vol 39, No. 7 [Suppl], 1990.)

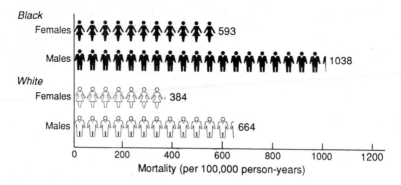

**Figure 4-14.** Age-adjusted mortality rates for all causes of death by race and gender in the United States, 1988. (Data from National Center for Health Statistics: Advance report of final mortality statistics, 1988. Monthly Vital Statistics Report. Vol 39, No. 7 [Suppl], 1990.)

BRFSS and the NHIS may be attributable to differences in sampling schemes, data collection methods, or both.

The NHIS prevalence estimates for cigarette smoking are shown by race and gender in Figure 4–22. These data indicate that cigarette use is most common among black males, followed by white males, black females, and white females, respectively. This pattern is consistent with the race and gender distribution of lung cancer mortality rates previously depicted in Figure 4–20. Although NHIS data indicate that the prevalence of cigarette smoking declined over the decade of the 1980s in all four race-gender groups, cigarette smoking remains the single most preventable cause of death in the United States. Progress towards meeting the national objective of reducing the prevalence of this behavior can be monitored through risk factor surveillance systems, such as the BRFSS and the NHIS.

## SUMMARY

In this chapter, lung cancer was used as a focus for consideration of the role of **surveillance** in epidemiology. Surveillance was defined as the detection of the occurrence of health-related events or exposures in a target population. Successful surveillance activities require continuity over time, standardized methodology, as well as timeliness of data collection and dissemination.

Surveillance data can be used in different ways, depending upon the type of information collected. Newly diagnosed persons with a disease can yield information on incidence rates; deaths from a disease can be used to describe mortality rates; and prevalence of risk factors can be used to predict future disease occurrence, or assess the status of prevention initiatives.

Surveillance activities in the United States related to lung cancer include collection of data on newly diagnosed persons (through population-based cancer registries), deaths (through death certificates), and prevalence of cigarette smoking (through population-based personal interview surveys).

The utility of **age adjustment** was demonstrated for the control of differences in underlying age structure when comparing summary rates of lung cancer incidence or mortality across population subgroups.

Key findings from surveillance related to lung cancer in the United States are listed below.

**Table 4–3.** Age-adjusted mortality rates per 100,000 person-years for the ten leading causes of death in the United States in 1988.[1]

| Rank | Cause of Death | Mortality Rate[2] |
|------|----------------|-------------------|
| 1 | Diseases of heart | 166.3 |
| 2 | Malignant neoplasms | 132.7 |
| 3 | Cerebrovascular disease | 29.7 |
| 4 | Unintentional injuries | 35.0 |
| 5 | Chronic obstructive pulmonary diseases | 19.4 |
| 6 | Pneumonia and influenza | 14.2 |
| 7 | Diabetes mellitus | 10.1 |
| 8 | Suicide | 11.4 |
| 9 | Chronic liver disease/cirrhosis | 9.0 |
| 10 | Nephritis/nephrotic syndrome/nephrosis | 4.8 |

[1] Data from CDC: Mortality patterns—United States, 1988. MMWR 1991;40:493.
[2] Directly adjusted to the 1940 population of the USA.

**(1)** Lung cancer has the second highest incidence, trailing only breast cancer. Malignancies of the lung are the leading cause of death from cancer.

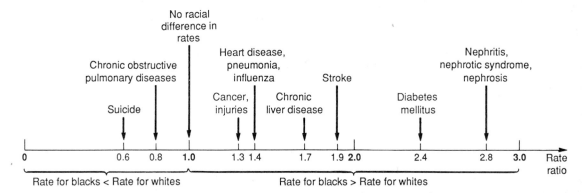

**Figure 4–15.** Black-to-white ratios of age-adjusted mortality rates for the ten leading causes of death in the United States, 1988. (Data from National Center for Health Statistics: Advance report of final mortality statistics, 1988. Monthly Vital Statistics Report. Vol 39, No. 7 [Suppl], 1990.)

**(2)** The incidence of lung cancer increases sharply between 30 and 70 years of age.

**(3)** The overall age-adjusted incidence rate of lung cancer is about 30% higher in blacks than whites. Contrast of age-adjusted mortality rates reveals a 55% higher rate among blacks.

**(4)** The age-adjusted mortality rate for lung cancer is about three-fourths of the corresponding incidence rate, indicating a high case fatality. Lung cancer age-adjusted mortality increased by about 20% in the decade of the 1980s.

**(5)** Age-adjusted mortality rates for lung cancer vary widely across states, as do the corresponding prevalences of cigarette smoking.

**(6)** The comparatively high age-adjusted mortality rate for lung cancer among black males is paralleled by a comparatively high prevalence of cigarette smoking.

Several features of the Patient Profile illustrate these descriptive patterns of lung cancer distribution. One, the patient was 68 years of age at presentation, a comparatively high-risk age for lung cancer occurrence. Two, she was a long-term cigarette smoker, thereby substantially increasing her risk of this disease. Three, the rapidity of her death following diagnosis is consistent with the high case fatality of this disease. With the generally poor treatment results for lung cancer, the greatest promise for controlling the impact of this disease is through preventing the initiation of cigarette smoking and encouraging current smokers to quit.

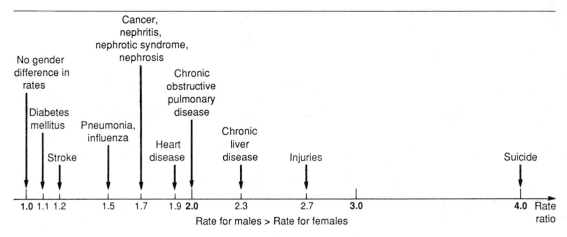

**Figure 4–16.** Male-to-female ratios of age-adjusted mortality rates for the ten leading causes of death in the United States, 1988. (Data from National Center for Health Statistics: Advance report of final mortality statistics, 1988. Monthly Vital Statistics Report. Vol 39, No. 7 [Suppl], 1990.)

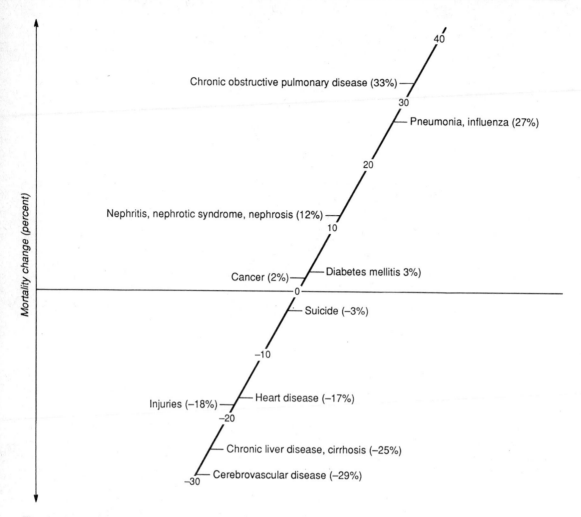

**Figure 4–17.** Ten-year percentage changes in age-adjusted mortality rates for leading causes of death in the United States, 1979–1988. (Data from National Center for Health Statistics: Advance report of final mortality statistics, 1988. Monthly Vital Statistics Report. Vol 39, No. 7 [Suppl], 1990.)

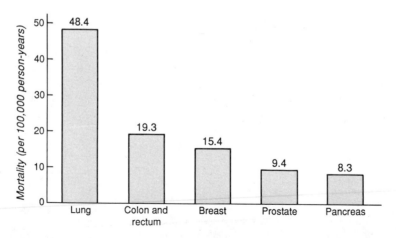

**Figure 4–18.** Age-adjusted mortality rates for the five leading forms of cancer in the United States, 1988. (Data from Ries LAG et al: *Cancer Statistics Review, 1973–88.* National Cancer Institute. NIH Publication No. 91–2789, 1991.)

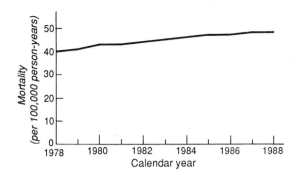

**Figure 4–19.** Age-adjusted mortality rates for lung cancer by calendar year in the United States, 1978–88. (Data from Ries LAG et al: *Cancer Statistics Review, 1973–88.* National Cancer Institute. NIH Publication No. 91–2789, 1991.)

## STUDY QUESTIONS

**Directions:** For each question, select the single best answer.

1. For which one of the following diseases is the age-adjusted mortality rate in the United States higher among whites than blacks?
   A. Nephritis/nephrotic syndrome/nephrosis
   B. Cerebrovascular disease
   C. Diabetes mellitus
   D. Suicide
   E. Chronic liver disease/cirrhosis

2. The leading cause of death in the United States is:
   A. Unintentional injuries
   B. Diseases of the heart
   C. Cerebrovascular diseases
   D. Malignant neoplasms
   E. Chronic obstructive pulmonary disease

3. In the United States, which one of the following causes of death has had the greatest increase in age-adjusted mortality rate during the past decade?
   A. Unintentional injuries
   B. Diseases of the heart
   C. Cerebrovascular diseases
   D. Malignant neoplasms
   E. Chronic obstructive pulmonary disease

4. Age-adjusted mortality from lung cancer in the United States is highest among which one of the following groups?
   A. Black males
   B. Black females
   C. White males
   D. White females

5. In the United States, which of the following primary anatomic sites is associated with the highest overall age-adjusted cancer incidence rate?
   A. Colon
   B. Lung
   C. Breast
   D. Prostate
   E. Pancreas

6. In the United States, cancer in which of the following organs results in the highest overall age-adjusted mortality rate?
   A. Colon
   B. Lung
   C. Breast
   D. Prostate
   E. Pancreas

7. In the United States, which of the following causes of death has the LEAST gender differential in age-adjusted mortality?
   A. Unintentional injuries
   B. Chronic obstructive pulmonary disease
   C. Suicide
   D. Diabetes mellitus
   E. Diseases of the heart

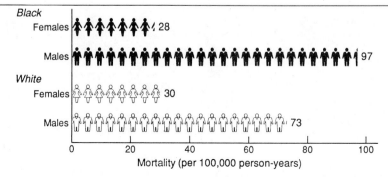

**Figure 4–20.** Age-adjusted mortality rates for lung cancer by race and gender in the United States, 1988. (Data from Ries LAG et al: *Cancer Statistics Review, 1973–88.* National Cancer Institute. NIH Publication No. 91–2789, 1991.)

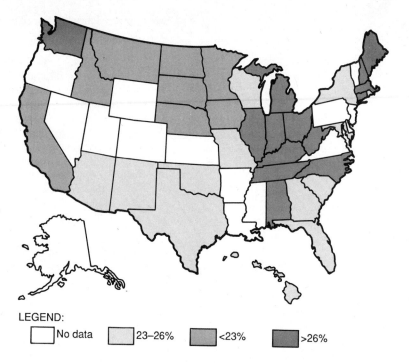

**Figure 4–21.** Prevalence of cigarette smoking, by state, United States, 1988. Unshaded areas represent states that did not participate in the Behavioral Risk Factor Surveillance System. (Data from CDC: Behavioral risk factor surveillance, 1988. MMWR 1990;39:(SS-2):1.)

8. Which of the following age groups (in years) has the highest incidence rate of lung cancer?
   A. 20–29
   B. 30–39
   C. 40–49
   D. 50–59
   E. 60–69

9. The prevalence of cigarette smoking in the United States is highest in which of the following groups?
   A. Black males
   B. Black females

C. White males
D. White females

10. The male-to-female ratio of age-adjusted mortality rates in the United States for pneumonia and influenza is 1.7. This means that compared to the age-adjusted mortality rate for females, the rate for males is:
   A. 7% higher
   B. 17% higher
   C. 70% higher
   D. 17% lower
   E. 70% lower

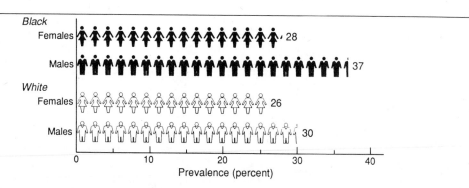

**Figure 4–22.** Prevalence of cigarette smoking in the United States by race and gender, 1988. (Data from CDC: Cigarette smoking among adults–United States, 1988. MMWR 1990;40:757.)

## FURTHER READING

Thacker SB, Berkelman RL: Public health surveillance in the United States. Epidemiol Rev 1988;10:164.

## REFERENCES

### Introduction
Berkelman RL, Buehler JW: Surveillance. In: *Oxford Textbook of Public Health,* 2nd ed. Vol 2. Holland WW, Detels R, Knox G (editors). Oxford Univ Press, 1991.

### Surveillance of New Diagnoses
Ries LAG et al: *Cancer Statistics Review, 1973–88.* National Cancer Institute. NIH Publication No. 91–2789, 1991.

### Age Adjustment
Dawson-Saunders B, Trapp RG: *Basic and Clinical Biostatistics.* Appleton & Lange, 1990.

### Mortality Patterns
National Center for Health Statistics: Advance report of final mortality statistics, 1988. Monthly Vital Statistics Report. Vol 39, No. 7 (Suppl), 1990.

### Surveillance of Risk Factors
CDC: Behavioral risk factor surveillance, 1988. MMWR 1990;30(SS-2):1.
CDC: Cigarette smoking among adults–United States, 1988. MMWR 1991;40:757.

# 5

# Disease Outbreaks

## PATIENT PROFILE

*A 23-year-old male student presented at 10:30 PM on January 17 at the college infirmary complaining of a sudden onset of abdominal cramping, nausea, and diarrhea. Although the patient was not in severe distress and had no fever or vomiting, he was weak. A number of other students, all with the same symptoms, visited the college infirmary over the next 20 hours. All patients were treated with bed rest and fluid replacement therapy. They recovered fully within 24 hours of the onset of illness.*

## INTRODUCTION

The concept of an epidemic as a dramatic rise in the occurrence of a disease was introduced in Chapter 3. When an epidemic occurs suddenly and in a relatively limited geographic area, it is described as a **disease outbreak.** The emergence of a disease outbreak requires immediate action in order to determine the origin of the problem, and ultimately, to prevent other persons from becoming affected.

In many outbreak situations, distinctive clinical features of the affected individuals may suggest the underlying cause (sometimes termed pathogen). A working hypothesis can lead to prompt identification of the causal agent and implementation of control measures. Ideally, the choice of control strategy is predicated upon knowledge of the source of the causal agent and how it is spread.

In other circumstances, however, the clinical features of affected individuals do not suggest a particular pathogen. An urgent response is required, although the investigator does not yet have a specific working hypothesis about the cause. Consequently, the first phase of investigation involves the collection of basic descriptive information in order to better characterize the illness and its pattern of occurrence. With this background descriptive data in hand, a hypothesis can be generated and then specific analytical studies can be designed to identify the causal factor.

The development and maintenance of a disease outbreak typically requires each of the following three characteristics: (1) the presence of a pathogen in sufficient quantities to affect multiple persons, (2) an appropriate mode of transmitting the pathogen to susceptible persons, and (3) an adequate pool of susceptible persons who are exposed to the pathogen. These three features are presented schematically in Figure 5–1.

Some outbreaks are self-limited and terminate without any intervention. In other situations, however, the outbreak will continue unless action is taken to prevent further spread. An effective control strategy should address one or more of the three conditions necessary for an epidemic. Specifically, the following interventions could terminate an outbreak:

- Removal or elimination of the source of the pathogen
- Blockage of the transmission process
- Elimination of susceptibility (eg, through vaccination or medication)

Epidemiologists often distinguish between two primary modes of transmission in acute outbreaks of disease: (1) **person-to-person** spread, and (2) **common-source** exposure. As the name implies, person-to-person spread occurs when the causal agent is transmitted from one individual to another. As described in Chapter 3, tuberculosis is a disease that is propagated in this manner, with the pathogen conveyed from an infectious person to a susceptible individual via airborne particles. The investigation of an outbreak of tuberculosis is likely to reveal an initial (or index) case and a number of subsequent cases that develop among the close contacts of the infectious person. An effective control strategy would involve isolation of the index case until that individual is no longer infectious, treatment of the index case with antibiotics to prevent further transmission, and preventive antibiotic therapy for infected close contacts.

A common-source exposure occurs when the causal agent is transmitted to affected individuals by some shared feature of the environment. For example, contaminated food can be the source of pathogenic bacteria for persons who ingest the food. Appropriate control measures for this type of outbreak would involve removal of the contaminated food as well as review of food preparation practices in order to prevent future outbreaks. Common-source outbreaks are not limited to infectious pathogens. For

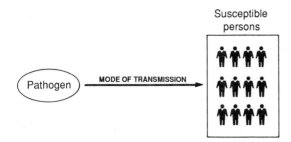

Susceptible persons

Pathogen — MODE OF TRANSMISSION →

**Figure 5–1.** Schematic representation of factors required for the development and maintenance of a disease outbreak.

example, chemical contamination of shared food, air, or water can result in an outbreak of disease.

Outbreaks of disease are fairly common and not all of these episodes can be investigated. In deciding whether an investigation is warranted, it is useful to consider the following factors:

- Apparent number of persons affected
- Presence of unusual or severe clinical symptoms
- Lack of an obvious explanation for disease occurrence
- Perceived need to implement control measures
- Level of public concern
- Potential for contributing to medical knowledge

The situation depicted in the Patient Profile did not involve a life-threatening condition, and the symptoms were rather typical of an acute gastrointestinal illness. On the basis of these criteria, an investigation of this outbreak would not be justified. On the other hand, a relatively large number of individuals were affected, the cause was uncertain, and members of this college community were concerned about further spread of the epidemic. With these circumstances in mind, an investigation of the outbreak was undertaken.

## THE EPIDEMIC

This epidemic of apparent gastroenteritis occurred on the campus of a liberal arts college in the northeastern United States. The temporal association of cases led to the working hypothesis that this epidemic was due to a microbial pathogen from a common source. It was suspected that there was one vehicle for transmission of the disease agent and, since the epidemic quickly peaked in time, that the vehicle was quickly exhausted or removed. The epidemic was investigated by public health authorities.

## THE INVESTIGATION

Existing information was gathered quickly, first at the infirmary and then at the college administration office. The index case presented to the infirmary at 10:30 PM on January 17, and by 8 PM on January 18, a total of 47 affected students were examined. A quantitative measure of the extent of an outbreak is the **attack rate** (*AR*). The *AR* rate is calculated using the following equation:

$$\text{Attack rate } (AR) = \frac{\text{Number of new cases}}{\text{Persons at risk}} \times 100$$

Note that the *AR* is a measure of risk, as defined in Chapter 2. Accordingly, a period of time must be specified in the estimation of an *AR*.

Knowledge that the college enrollment was 1164 allows the *AR* for the gastrointestinal disease outbreak to be calculated. The *AR* for the period from 10:30 PM January 17 to 8 PM January 18 was:

$$\text{Attack rate}_{\text{(all students)}} = \frac{47}{1164} \times 100 = 4.0\%$$

It readily was apparent, however, that the population at risk could be defined more narrowly because all students who reported to the infirmary lived in dormitories on campus, but only about two-thirds of all enrolled students lived in dormitories. In other words, the one-third of students who lived outside of dormitories did not appear to be at risk of disease. Since these students were not entered into the numerator of the equation, their inclusion in the denominator makes the calculation potentially misleading. A more precise estimate of the *AR*, based upon the 756 students at risk in the dormitories was:

$$\text{Attack rate}_{\text{(dorm residents)}} = \frac{47}{756} \times 100 = 6.2\%$$

By defining the population at risk more precisely, the estimated *AR* increased by more than 50%.

Since the patients' dormitories were recorded on infirmary records, the *AR*s could be calculated by dormitory and by gender (dormitories were separated by gender). These data are presented in Table 5–1. The difference in the *AR*s was striking and clearly suggested that the residents of two dormitories (1 and 12) were at greater risk than residents of the other 12 dormitories. A combined *AR* for these two dormitories can be contrasted with the other 12 dormitories as follows:

$$\text{Attack rate}_{\text{(dorms 1, 12)}} = \frac{(19 + 13)}{(80 + 62)} \times 100 = 22.5\%$$

The *AR* for the remaining 12 dormitories was:

$$\text{Attack rate}_{\text{(remaining dorms)}} = \frac{(47 - 32)}{(756 - 142)} \times 100$$
$$= \frac{15}{614} \times 100 = 2.4\%$$

**Table 5–1.** The dormitory of residence of the 47 known cases and the attack rate, as well as the population and gender of the occupants of each dormitory.

| Dormitory | Gender | Population at Risk | Number of Cases | Attack Rate (AR) (%) |
|---|---|---|---|---|
| 1 | F | 80 | 19 | 23.8 |
| 2 | F | 62 | 2 | 3.2 |
| 3 | F | 89 | 0 | 0 |
| 4 | F | 61 | 1 | 1.6 |
| 5 | F | 53 | 5 | 9.4 |
| 6 | M | 35 | 0 | 0 |
| 7 | M | 63 | 0 | 0 |
| 8 | F | 103 | 4 | 3.9 |
| 9 | M | 35 | 1 | 2.9 |
| 10 | M | 37 | 0 | 0 |
| 11 | F | 34 | 1 | 2.9 |
| 12 | M | 62 | 13 | 21.0 |
| 13 | M | 32 | 1 | 3.1 |
| 14 | M | 10 | 0 | 0 |
| Total | — | 756 | 47 | 6.2 |

A ratio of these attack rates may be calculated as follows:

$$\text{Risk ratio} = \frac{AR_{(\text{dorms 1, 12})}}{AR_{(\text{remaining dorms})}} = \frac{22.5\%}{2.4\%} = 9.4$$

This risk ratio means that the $AR$ in dormitories 1 and 12 was 9.4 times greater than in the remaining 12 dormitories.

A different ratio could be constructed using just the number of cases. Such a ratio would be 32 cases (dormitories 1 and 12) divided by the 15 cases in the remaining 12 dormitories. This ratio is 32/15, or 2.1. It should be clear, however, that this latter ratio is not an appropriate comparison since it does not take into account the differing sizes of the populations at risk in the dormitories. There were only one-fourth as many students at risk in dormitories 1 and 12, and so one would not expect the same number of cases to occur in these two dormitories as occurred in the other 12 dormitories. If the residents of dormitories 1 and 12 experienced the same risk as other dormitory residents, then the expected number of cases in dormitories 1 and 12 would be:

**Expected cases**$_{(\text{dorms 1, 12})}$

$= \textbf{Students at risk}_{(\text{dorms 1, 12})} \times \textbf{AR}_{(\text{remaining dorms})}$

$= 142 \times \dfrac{15}{614} = 3.5$

The frequency data in Table 5–1 also can be used to calculate rates by gender. For males, the $AR$ was:

$$AR_{(\text{males})} = \frac{(1 + 13 + 1)}{(35 + 63 + 35 + 37 + 62 + 32 + 10)} \times 100$$

$$= \frac{15}{274} \times 100 = 5.5\%$$

A similar calculation for females yielded an $AR$ of 6.6%. The ratio of attack rates for females-to-males was 1.2, indicating that there was not much gender difference in risk of acquiring this disease.

Visits to some of the campus dormitories by the investigators soon revealed that not all students who became ill had visited the infirmary. Thus, it became important to obtain additional data regarding the nature and extent of the outbreak, which, it was hoped, would be less biased by differences in care-seeking behavior. Questionnaires were prepared and distributed by hand to all students living in seven dormitories chosen to provide a representative sample of the student population. The results from this survey are presented in Table 5–2. A different picture of this epidemic emerged from these results. The overall $AR$ now could be calculated as:

$$\text{Attack rate} = \frac{110}{304} \times 100 = 36.2\%$$

Note that the denominator for this $AR$ was 304, the number of returned questionnaires, not 411, the total number of eligible students. Since nonrespondents could not be classified according to disease status (in the numerator of the $AR$ calculation), their inclusion

**Table 5–2.** Responses to the questionnaire survey by dormitory.[1]

| Dormitory | Population | Questionnaires Returned | | Number of ill Students |
|---|---|---|---|---|
| | | Number | Percent | |
| 5 | 53 | 49 | 92.5 | 13 |
| 6 | 35 | 26 | 74.3 | 13 |
| 7 | 63 | 28 | 44.4 | 15 |
| 8 | 103 | 65 | 63.1 | 21 |
| 9 | 35 | 19 | 54.3 | 5 |
| 12 | 62 | 44 | 71.0 | 22 |
| Nurses' residence[2] | 60 | 60 | 100 | 17 |
| Unidentified[3] | — | 13 | — | 4 |
| Total | 411 | 304 | 74.0 | 110 |

[1] Dormitories 1–4, 10, 11, 13, and 14 were not surveyed.
[2] Nurses' dormitory located off campus.
[3] Dormitory of residence not entered on 13 questionnaires.

in the denominator makes the *AR* calculation invalid. In the initial infirmary data, the *AR*s for dormitories 6 and 12 were 0 and 21%, respectively. From the survey responses, however, these dormitories did not appear to have different *AR*s:

$$AR_{(dorm\ 6)} = \frac{13}{26} \times 100 = 50\%$$

$$AR_{(dorm\ 12)} = \frac{22}{44} \times 100 = 50\%$$

In other words, the infirmary records and the questionnaire data gave two very different perspectives on the distribution of the outbreak by place of residence. The explanation for this discrepancy was not immediately apparent, but could have reflected differences in approaches to data collection. The infirmary data were useful in the initial phase of investigation because they were readily available. On the other hand, these data could have been influenced by various factors, such as variation in the severity of illness and care-seeking behavior. The student survey tended to avoid these problems.

The true *AR* of gastroenteritis on campus was not known. The best estimate was 36.2%, as determined from the student survey, but this *AR* could have been incorrect since only 74% of the survey questionnaires were returned (see Table 5–2). If the illness experience of the nonrespondents differed appreciably from the three-fourths of students who responded, then the estimated *AR* could have been incorrect. It is possible, for example, that students who were not affected by the illness were less motivated to respond to the survey. Under these circumstances, the calculated *AR* of 36.2% would be higher than the true *AR* for all students. The extent to which the estimated and true *AR* differed reflects **bias,** or lack of validity. Another potential source of bias could have arisen in the selection of the dormitories to be surveyed. To the extent that these dormitories were systematically different from the remaining nonsurveyed dormitories, then bias could have been introduced into the estimation of the true *AR*. Furthermore, if students misreported

their illness experience, either intentionally or nonintentionally, then a distorted pattern of the outbreak could have emerged.

The concept of bias will be discussed at length in Chapter 10. Suffice it to say that it is desirable to minimize the amount of bias in any study. In order to reduce the potential for bias in the present context, the amount of missing information must be minimized. Since the investigators could not force students to respond, it would be unrealistic to expect complete participation. Nevertheless, strategies could be used to increase the response level by various techniques, such as the use of reminders and peer support. The pattern of response rates shown in Table 5–2 was clearly nonrandom, with particularly low response levels in dormitories 7, 8, and 9. Focused efforts to increase participation among residents of those dormitories might have helped to increase confidence in the validity of findings.

Several factors could explain why the *AR*s estimated from infirmary records were low. Some students may have experienced mild illness that did not require medical attention, and others may have sought care elsewhere. It also was discovered that dormitories 1 and 12, which initially appeared to have the highest *AR*s, were located adjacent to the infirmary, and access to this facility was more convenient for residents of these dormitories.

The survey data indicated a much higher *AR* and more widespread nature of the disease than originally suspected; in fact, more than one-third of all students appeared to be involved. In addition, the abrupt onset of disease and clustering of cases in time suggested a common-source exposure. Data collected during the survey indicated that no large gatherings of students, such as parties or sports events, had recently occurred. Attention then was directed at meals, since most students ate at the college cafeteria. Included in the survey were questions concerning the source of meals eaten on January 16 and 17. Information from the survey is summarized in Table 5–3. Data are presented in a format that is typical for food histories. *AR*s are presented for those who ate and those who did not eat each meal. For example, 152 students ate

**Table 5–3.** Analysis of meal-specific exposure histories of the respondents to the questionnaire.

| Meal | Students Who ATE Specific Meal | | | | Students Who DID NOT EAT Specific Meal | | | |
|---|---|---|---|---|---|---|---|---|
| | ill | Well | Total | AR (%) | ill | Well | Total | AR (%) |
| January 16 | | | | | | | | |
| Breakfast | 52 | 100 | 152 | 34.2 | 51 | 94 | 145 | 35.2 |
| Lunch | 89 | 150 | 239 | 37.2 | 20 | 44 | 64 | 31.3 |
| Dinner | 87 | 150 | 237 | 36.7 | 23 | 44 | 67 | 34.3 |
| January 17 | | | | | | | | |
| Breakfast | 56 | 105 | 161 | 34.8 | 42 | 89 | 131 | 32.1 |
| Lunch | 106 | 145 | 251 | 42.2 | 3 | 49 | 52 | 5.8 |
| Dinner | 78 | 130 | 208 | 37.5 | 31 | 64 | 95 | 32.6 |

breakfast on January 16, and of these, 52 reported that they became ill. Thus, the AR was (52/152) × 100 = 34.2%. ARs were calculated in a similar manner for all meals on these days.

The relationship between eating a particular meal and developing illness was assessed by contrasting ARs in those who ate and those who did not eat that meal. Most ARs, not surprisingly, were approximately 36%, with little difference between those who did or did not eat a particular meal. The exception was found for the January 17 lunch meal. A ratio of ARs (risk ratio) for eaters and noneaters of this meal was calculated as follows:

$$RR_{(1/17\ lunch)} = \frac{AR_{(1/17\ lunch\ eaters)}}{AR_{(1/17\ lunch\ noneaters)}} = \frac{42.2\%}{5.8\%} = 7.3$$

This risk ratio indicates that those who ate this meal were more than seven times as likely to become ill as those who did not eat this meal. Similar risk ratios were calculated for the other meals and were close to 1.0. For example, the risk ratio for dinner on January 17 was 37.5/32.6 = 1.2.

Having identified the meal at which the students most probably were exposed and knowing each student's time of onset of symptoms, it was possible to calculate the **incubation period,** in this case the time between eating the meal and the onset of symptoms, for 101 ill students. The distribution of these incubation periods is shown in Table 5–4 and presented graphically in Figures 5–2 and 5–3. In Figure 5–2, the number of cases that occurred is shown by time in hours between exposure and onset of illness. In Figure 5–3, the cumulative percentage distribution of cases is presented by incubation period. *The median incubation period is the time by which 50% of the cases have occurred.* The median incubation period in Figure 5–3 is 10 hours. A follow-up survey was directed at obtaining information about the noon meal of January 17. Data from the follow-up study are presented in Table 5–5.

In order to identify the food(s) responsible for the outbreak, dietary histories were analyzed. The questionnaires provided information about what particular foods 251 students ate at the noon meal on Friday, January 17. If students were uncertain about whether or not they ate the food in question, they were not

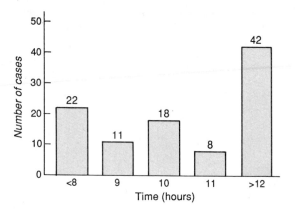

**Figure 5–2.** Distribution of number of cases by time from eating suspect meal to development of symptoms.

included in the analysis of that particular food. As a consequence, the total of those who ate and those who did not eat each specific item did not equal 251 for all items.

The ratios of ARs yielded values greater than 1.0 for certain items, indicating that the risk of illness was greater among students who ate that item than among those who did not eat the item. For other items the values were less than 1.0, indicating that risk of illness was lower among those who ate the item in question. For example, the risk ratio was 0.7 for fish chowder, 1.0 for fruit salad, and 8.0 for lamb stew pie. It was clear from these data that the risk ratio for illness was considerably higher for those who ate lamb stew pie than for those who did not. This information suggested that lamb stew pie was the most likely source of exposure to the pathogen. Further investigation of the preparation of the lamb stew pie indicated that it was prepared the previous day (January 16), refrigerated, and warmed on the morning it was served.

**Table 5–4.** Distribution of incubation periods.

| Incubation Period (Hours) | Number of Students | Cumulative Number of Students |
| --- | --- | --- |
| ≤8 | 22 | 22 |
| 9 | 11 | 33 |
| 10 | 18 | 51 |
| 11 | 8 | 59 |
| ≥12 | 42 | 101 |

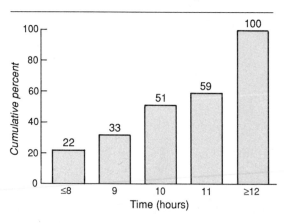

**Figure 5–3.** Cumulative percentage distribution of cases by time from eating suspect meal to development of symptoms.

**Table 5–5.** Food-specific histories of students who ate lunch at the college cafeteria on January 17.

| Food or Beverage | Students Who Ate Specific Food or Beverage | | | | Students Who Did Not Eat Specific Food or Beverage | | | |
|---|---|---|---|---|---|---|---|---|
| | ill | Well | Total | AR (%) | ill | Well | Total | AR (%) |
| Fish chowder | 16 | 36 | 52 | 30.8 | 87 | 103 | 190 | 45.8 |
| Lamb stew pie | 95 | 56 | 151 | 62.9 | 7 | 82 | 89 | 7.9 |
| Tuna noodle casserole | 12 | 57 | 69 | 17.4 | 92 | 80 | 172 | 53.5 |
| Pineapple Jell-O salad | 58 | 54 | 112 | 51.8 | 39 | 69 | 108 | 36.1 |
| Fruit salad | 32 | 39 | 71 | 45.1 | 63 | 82 | 145 | 43.4 |
| Cabbage salad | 4 | 5 | 9 | 44.4 | 95 | 126 | 221 | 43.0 |
| Plain Jell-O with vanilla sauce | 19 | 29 | 48 | 39.6 | 80 | 102 | 182 | 44.0 |
| Plain Jell-O without vanilla sauce | 62 | 77 | 139 | 44.6 | 39 | 56 | 95 | 41.1 |
| Milk | 91 | 127 | 218 | 41.7 | 12 | 13 | 25 | 48.0 |
| Coffee | 10 | 31 | 41 | 24.4 | 89 | 103 | 192 | 46.4 |
| Tea | 23 | 19 | 42 | 54.8 | 78 | 114 | 192 | 40.6 |

Although no specific laboratory studies were performed, the etiologic agent that caused this outbreak could be inferred from available information. The illness was marked by gastrointestinal symptoms of limited duration, usually without fever or vomiting; the median incubation period was 10 hours; and a meat dish was presumed to be the most likely source of the pathogen. Based upon these observations, the etiologic agent probably was *Clostridium perfringens*. When ingested from inadequately cooked foods, particularly stews, meats, or gravies, type A strains of this bacterium produce a toxin that causes gastrointestinal symptoms. The incubation period, which may range from 8–22 hours, is typically 10–12 hours. The absence of fever differentiated this particular gastrointestinal illness from shigellosis or salmonellosis, and the absence of vomiting distinguished this illness from food poisoning by staphylococcal bacteria or chemical agents.

Since *C perfringens* food poisoning does not involve person-to-person transmission, it is not necessary to isolate affected patients. Supportive treatment should include oral administration of fluids and electrolytes, or intravenous therapy in severe cases. Antibiotic treatment is not required. Taking measures to reduce bacterial proliferation in food sources can prevent outbreaks of *C perfringens* food poisoning. Thorough cooking of meats and stews at an adequate temperature is essential. Dividing stews into small cooking portions helps to ensure uniform heating and decreases the need to store and reheat leftovers.

## SUMMARY

The investigation of **disease outbreaks** (sudden and geographically limited epidemics) is an essential role of epidemiology. The primary goals of an outbreak investigation are the identification of the causal agent (pathogen) and the prevention of the development of further cases. The propagation of a disease outbreak requires a pathogen, a viable mode of transmission, and an adequate pool of susceptible persons. Elimination of one or more of these three components will terminate the outbreak. Two basic modes of transmission are **person-to-person** spread and **common-source** exposure. Infectious illnesses can be transmitted by either mode, whereas noninfectious environmental pathogens more typically produce disease outbreaks through a common-source transmission.

Not all disease outbreaks warrant investigation. The decision to investigate an outbreak typically is based upon the severity of illness, the number of affected persons, uncertainty about the pathogen, and the perceived need to control further spread of the disease. Investigations typically are conducted by local, state, or federal public health officials.

In this chapter, the principles and methods of outbreak investigation were illustrated by the evaluation of an episode of food poisoning on a college campus. This outbreak came to attention because almost 50 students sought medical attention for acute gastrointestinal symptoms in a period of less than 24 hours.

A measure of the risk of developing the illness in question over a specified period of time is the **attack rate** (*AR*). Based upon infirmary records, the *AR* among all students was estimated to be 4%, but among those residing in dormitories, the estimated *AR* was 6%. The *AR* did not differ by gender, but students residing at two dormitories had higher *AR*s than residents of the other 12 dormitories.

In order to collect more detailed, and perhaps more complete, information than could be obtained from infirmary records, a survey was performed of residents of a representative sample of dormitories. The survey results indicated a much higher *AR* for dormitory residents (36%) than had been estimated from infirmary records (6%). The possibility of **bias** (systematic error) in both estimates must be considered. Nevertheless, the results of the survey suggested that the outbreak was widespread among dormitory residents and also indicated that the prior definition of high-risk dormitories based upon infirmary records might be inaccurate.

Comparison of *AR*s for persons who ate and did not eat specific foods indicated a strong association between eating a particular food and risk of the gastrointestinal illness. The distribution of times from ingestion to the onset of symptoms (incubation period) revealed a median time interval of about 10 hours. A follow-up survey revealed that lamb stew pie was the most suspect common-source exposure for this outbreak.

Although cultures of the foods and specimens from affected individuals were not obtained, the nature of the symptoms, the median incubation period, and the presumed source of exposure implicated *Clostridium perfringens* as the pathogen. Knowledge of the factors that contribute to the proliferation and transmission of this bacteria were used to control this outbreak and could be used to prevent similar episodes in the future.

## STUDY QUESTIONS

**Directions:** For each question, select the single best answer.

**Questions 1–2.** During an 8-hour work shift at a corporate headquarters building, 30 employees (20 females and ten males) visited the company's physician with complaints of nausea, vomiting, headaches, and dizziness. All affected individuals responded to supportive treatment and were sent home. In order to search for possible causes of the outbreak, the physician performed an investigation.

1. If 600 persons worked in the building, then the attack rate was:
   A. 3%
   B. 5%
   C. 10%
   D. 20%
   E. 30%

2. If 400 females and 200 males worked in the building, the male-to-female risk ratio was:
   A. 0.3
   B. 0.5
   C. 1.0
   D. 2.0
   E. 3.0

**Questions 3–5.** The distribution of cases and population at risk is shown by floor of the building in Table 5–6.

3. The floor with the highest risk of disease was:
   A. A
   B. B
   C. C
   D. D
   E. E

4. The risk for workers on the high-risk floor was how many times greater than the average risk among all workers?
   A. 1
   B. 2
   C. 3
   D. 4
   E. 5

5. If the average risk among all workers was applied to the number of workers on the high-risk floor, the expected number of cases on that floor would have been:
   A. 1
   B. 2
   C. 3
   D. 4
   E. 5

**Questions 6–8.** A survey of all workers was conducted to determine whether other persons were affected beyond those who sought care at the physician's office. All 600 employees were surveyed, and 400 questionnaires were completed and returned. A total of 80 persons reported symptoms consistent with the syndrome observed among workers who sought medical attention.

6. The response rate to the questionnaire was:
   A. 5.0%
   B. 7.5%
   C. 20.0%
   D. 37.5%
   E. 67.0%

7. Based on the survey data, the attack rate was:
   A. 5.0%
   B. 7.5%

**Table 5–6.** Distribution of cases and population at risk by floor of the office building.

| Floor | Number of Cases | Persons at Risk |
|-------|-----------------|-----------------|
| A | 4 | 20 |
| B | 7 | 155 |
| C | 6 | 135 |
| D | 8 | 180 |
| E | 5 | 110 |
| Total | 30 | 600 |

C. 20.0%
D. 37.5%
E. 67.0%

8. The percentage of affected individuals who sought medical care was:
   A. 5.0%
   B. 7.5%
   C. 20.0%
   D. 37.5%
   E. 67.0%

**Questions 9–10.** Based upon responses to the survey, the exposure most strongly associated with the development of illness was drinking from a water cooler on the entrance level of the building. The cumulative percentage distribution of times from first drinking from the water cooler that day to the development of symptoms is shown in Figure 5–4.

9. From this graph, the median incubation period in hours was:
   A. 1
   B. 2
   C. 3
   D. 4
   E. 5

10. Factors that suggested a common-source exposure included all of the following EXCEPT

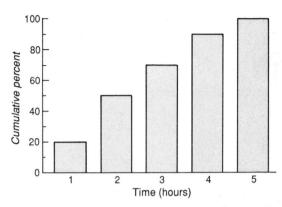

**Figure 5–4.** Cumulative percentage distribution of cases by time from first drinking from water cooler to onset of illness.

A. Tight clustering of cases in time of onset
B. No more than average risk among office mates of cases
C. Lack of similar illnesses among family members of cases
D. Lack of further cases when the water cooler was removed
E. Large number of affected persons

## FURTHER READING

Goodman RA, Buehler JW, Koplan JP: The epidemiologic field investigation: Science and judgment in public health practice. Am J Epidemiol 1990:132:9.

## REFERENCES

Gregg MB, Parsonnet J: The principles of an epidemic field investigation. In: *Oxford Textbook of Public Health,* 2nd ed, Vol 2. Holland WW, Detels R, Knox G (editors). Oxford Univ Press, 1991.

Kelsey JL, Thompson WD, Evans AS: Epidemic investigation. In: *Methods in Observational Epidemiology.* Oxford Univ Press, 1986.

# 6

# Diagnostic Testing

## PATIENT PROFILE

*A 54-year-old high school teacher visited her family practitioner for an annual checkup. She reported no illnesses during the preceding year, felt well, and had no complaints. The hot flashes she had experienced a year ago had cleared up without treatment. The physician performed a physical examination, comprising breast, pelvic (including a Papanicolaou smear), and rectal examinations; all were unremarkable. The physician recommended that the patient have a mammogram, which was scheduled one week later.*

*The results of the mammogram were not normal, and the radiologist suggested that a breast biopsy be performed. The family practitioner notified the patient of the abnormal mammogram and referred her to a surgeon, who concurred that physical examination of the breast was normal. Based upon the mammographic abnormality, however, the surgeon and the radiologist agreed that fine needle aspiration (FNA) of the abnormal breast under radiologic guidance was indicated. Evaluation of the FNA specimen by a pathologist revealed cancer cells, and the patient was scheduled for further surgery the following week.*

## CLINICAL REASONING

The practice of clinical medicine is the artful application of science. There was a seemingly straightforward chain of decisions by the physicians in the Patient Profile that ultimately lead to the diagnosis of breast cancer and subsequent treatment. In practice, however, the process of clinical reasoning can be extremely complex. Each of the decisions made by the clinicians in the Patient Profile included the possibility that information was incorrect. Sir William Osler eloquently described the difficulties of clinical decision making in 1921:

> The problems of disease are more complicated and difficult than any others with which the trained mind has to grapple. . .Variability is the law of life. As no two faces are the same, so no two bodies are alike, and no two individuals react alike and behave alike under the abnormal conditions which we know as disease. This is the

fundamental difficulty in the education of the physician, and one which he [or she] may never grasp. . ."Probability is the guide of life."

The clinical decision-making process is based on probability. For example, in the Patient Profile, the clinician knew that a 54-year-old woman with a normal breast examination had a low probability of having breast cancer ($\approx 0.3\%$). An abnormal screening mammogram increased the likelihood of breast cancer to perhaps 13%. The radiologist may have predicted a slightly lower or higher probability of breast cancer based upon the particular mammographic findings. A positive FNA test increased the probability of breast cancer to about 64%. Again, based upon the particulars of this patient's FNA specimen, such as the appearance of the nucleus or the nuclear/cytoplasmic ratio, the estimate of the probability of breast cancer after the FNA may have been slightly more or less than 64%. Furthermore, different pathologists may reach different conclusions when interpreting the same microscopic specimen, ie, some pathologists may state that cancer cells are definitely present, while others may report that the specimen is suspicious for cancer.

Figure 6–1 is a diagrammatic representation of the diagnostic process that ultimately leads to a diagnosis of breast cancer in the Patient Profile. The likelihood of a particular disease at any point in time is given on the horizontal axis. At the far left, the probability of disease is 0, and at the far right, the probability of disease is 100%. The likelihood of disease moves toward 0 or 100% based upon each new meaningful piece of information. In the Patient Profile, the probability of breast cancer for the patient increased from close to 0 to almost 67% during the diagnostic workup. *The purpose of a diagnostic test is to move the estimated probability of disease toward either end of the probability scale,* thereby providing information that will alter subsequent diagnostic or treatment plans. When the estimated probability of a disease is close to 0, the disease can be ruled out. When the estimated likelihood of a disease is close to 100%, disease is confirmed.

Although diagnostic procedures, such as x-rays or biopsies, often are thought of as laboratory tests, almost all approaches to gathering clinical information

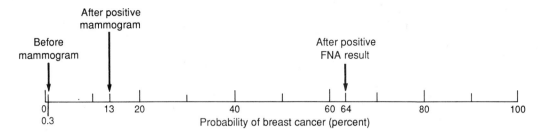

**Figure 6–1.** Schematic diagram of the estimated probabilities of breast cancer in a 54-year-old woman without a palpable breast mass: (1) before a mammogram, (2) after a positive mammogram, and (3) following a positive FNA test result.

can be regarded as tests. A patient's responses to questions during a history or the presence or absence of physical findings influences the clinician's estimation of the probability of the particular disease. In the Patient Profile, if the patient's sister and mother previously were diagnosed with breast cancer, then the patient's likelihood of having breast cancer prior to any tests could have been as high as 1%. If a palpable breast lump was present on physical examination, then the likelihood of cancer could have been estimated to be 20–40% prior to the mammogram. Experienced diagnosticians typically form hypotheses early in a patient encounter and then direct the history and physical examination in an effort to refine the estimated probabilities of a relatively small number of diseases.

Tests may be performed for many reasons. In the preceding discussion, attention was focused on determining the probability that a disease was present. Tests also may be used to assess the severity of an illness, predict disease outcome, or monitor response to therapy. Regardless of the purpose of a test, it is important to remember that the test is used to estimate probability of an outcome.

## SENSITIVITY AND SPECIFICITY

In a perfect world, medical tests would always be correct. For example, women could undergo a diagnostic test with no side effects that would unequivocally determine whether or not breast cancer was present. A positive test result would indicate that cancer was present and a negative test result would indicate that the disease was absent. In reality, however, every test is fallible.

Consider a test that has only positive or negative results. After the test is performed, one of four possible scenarios will occur, as demonstrated in Figure 6–2. For the purposes of this discussion, "true" disease status is determined by the most definitive diagnostic method, referred to as a "gold standard." For example, the gold standard for breast cancer diagnosis might be histopathologic confirmation of cancer in a surgical specimen. In cell *a* of Figure 6–2, the dis-

ease of interest is present and the test result is positive, or true-positive. In cell *d*, the disease is absent and the test is negative, or true-negative. In both of these cells, the test result agrees with the actual disease status. Cell *b* represents those persons without disease who have a positive test result. Since these test results incorrectly suggest that disease is present, they are considered to be false-positives. Those persons in cell *c* have the disease but have negative test results. These results are designated false-negatives because they incorrectly suggest that disease is absent.

Any diagnostic test can be evaluated in this manner. The first step in the evaluation of a test is how to determine the "true" disease status. For the FNA test, we could compare results obtained from FNA to the results obtained if every woman subsequently underwent a surgical excisional biopsy procedure. This procedure, the gold standard, is considered to represent the true disease status.

Just such a comparison of FNA results against excisional biopsy was made in 114 consecutive women with normal physical examinations and abnormal mammograms who received a FNA followed by a surgical excisional biopsy of the same breast (Bibbo et al, 1988). The results of the comparison are given in Figure 6–3.

**Sensitivity** and **specificity** are two terms used to describe the performance of the FNA test relative to the surgical excisional biopsy. *The sensitivity of a test is defined as the percentage of persons with the dis-*

| | "Truth" | |
|---|---|---|
| | Disease | No disease |
| **Test result**<br>Positive | **a**<br>True-positive | **b**<br>False-positive |
| Negative | **c**<br>False-negative | **d**<br>True-negative |

**Figure 6–2.** Format for comparison of results of a diagnostic test against the "true" disease status.

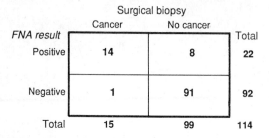

Surgical biopsy

| FNA result | Cancer | No cancer | Total |
|---|---|---|---|
| Positive | 14 | 8 | 22 |
| Negative | 1 | 91 | 92 |
| Total | 15 | 99 | 114 |

**Figure 6–3.** Comparison of FNA test results with findings from surgical excisional biopsies in women without palpable breast masses. (Data reproduced, with permission, from Bibbo M et al: Stereotaxic fine needle aspiration cytology of clinically occult malignant and premalignant breast lesions. Acta Cytol 1988;32:193.)

*ease of interest who have positive test results.* Sensitivity is calculated as follows:

$$\text{Sensitivity} = \frac{\text{True-positives}}{\text{True-positives + False-negatives}} \times 100$$

$$= \frac{a}{a + c} \times 100$$

Substituting data from Figure 6–3, the sensitivity of the FNA test is:

$$\text{Sensitivity} = \frac{\text{True-positives}}{\text{True-positives + False-negatives}} \times 100$$

$$= \frac{14}{14 + 1} \times 100 = 93\%$$

The greater the sensitivity of a test, the more likely that the test will detect persons with the disease of interest. For the FNA test, 93% of all the patients with breast cancer had positive FNA test results. Tests with great sensitivity are useful clinically to rule out a disease. That is, a negative result would virtually exclude the possibility that the patient has the disease of interest.

*Specificity is defined as the percentage of persons without the disease of interest who have negative test results.* Specificity is calculated as follows:

$$\text{Specificity} = \frac{\text{True-negatives}}{\text{True-negatives + False-positives}} \times 100$$

$$= \frac{d}{b + d} \times 100$$

Substituting data from Figure 6–3, the specificity of the FNA test is:

$$\text{Specificity} = \frac{\text{True-negatives}}{\text{True-negatives + False-positives}} \times 100$$

$$= \frac{91}{91 + 8} \times 100 = 92\%$$

The greater the specificity, the more likely that persons without the disease of interest will be excluded by the test. Very specific tests often are used to confirm the presence of a disease. If the test is highly specific, a positive test result would strongly implicate the disease of interest.

## POSITIVE AND NEGATIVE PREDICTIVE VALUE

Sensitivity and specificity are descriptors of the accuracy of a test. Two measure that directly address the estimation of probability of disease are the **positive predictive value (PV⁺)** and the **negative predictive value (PV⁻)**. *The PV⁺ is defined as the percentage of persons with positive test results who actually have the disease of interest.* The PV⁺ therefore, allows one to estimate how likely it is that the disease of interest is present if the test is positive. Referring again to Figure 6–2, the PV⁺ is calculated as follows:

$$\text{PV}^+ = \frac{\text{True-positives}}{\text{True-positives + False-positives}} \times 100$$

$$= \frac{a}{a + b} \times 100$$

The PV⁺ is the percentage of persons who both have the disease and a positive test result among all persons with positive test results. The calculation of the PV⁺ for the FNA test described in Figure 6–3 is:

$$\text{PV}^+ = \frac{\text{True-positives}}{\text{True-positives + False-negatives}} \times 100$$

$$= \frac{14}{14 + 8} \times 100 = 64\%$$

The average probability of breast cancer among women in this sample prior to the FNA test was 15 affected women out of 114 total women, or 13%. After the FNA test, the probability of breast cancer for a woman with a positive test result increased to 64%.

*The PV⁻ is the probability of breast cancer being absent if the FNA is negative.* The general formula for the calculation of PV⁻ is:

$$\text{PV}^- = \frac{\text{True-negatives}}{\text{True-negatives + False-negatives}} \times 100$$

$$= \frac{d}{c + d} \times 100$$

For the FNA test data in Figure 6–3, the PV⁻ is:

$$PV^- = \frac{\text{True-negatives}}{\text{True-negatives} + \text{False-negatives}} \times 100$$

$$= \frac{91}{1 + 91} \times 100 = 99\%$$

Before the FNA test was performed, the average likelihood of not having breast cancer among women in this sample was 99 unaffected women out of 114 total women, or 87%. After a negative FNA test result, the probability of not having breast cancer increased to 99%.

Now that the post-FNA probability of disease has been calculated for either a positive or negative test result, one can consider the usefulness of the FNA test for a patient with a nonpalpable breast lesion. A positive test result increased the probability of breast cancer from 13% to 64%. Whether the probability of breast cancer is 13% or 64%, further workup or treatment is indicated. Both before and after a positive FNA test result, the clinician would feel that breast cancer was too likely not to proceed with a test such as a surgical biopsy, which would provide the most definitive diagnosis.

A negative test result, however, would reduce the probability of breast cancer being present to 1%

(100% − PV⁻ = 1%). One could choose to defer surgical biopsy and repeat mammographic examinations in several months on women with abnormal mammograms but normal FNAs, accepting a one in 100 risk of delayed treatment of an existing cancer. A more aggressive approach would be to perform a surgical biopsy on every woman with an abnormal mammogram. The basis of this decision would be that a probability of breast cancer of 1% is too high *not* to proceed with a surgical biopsy. The advantage of performing an FNA on patients with abnormal mammograms is that the vast majority of these women could be spared the increased morbidity and expense associated with a surgical biopsy.

In addition to recognizing that all tests are fallible, it is important to appreciate that the usefulness of a test changes as the clinical situation changes. Specifically, the pretest probability of disease in an individual, or the prevalence of disease in a population, greatly influences the predictive value. The concept of variable test performance can be illustrated by comparing the use of FNA in women with mammographically detected breast lesions without palpable breast masses to the use of FNA test in women with breast masses found on physical examination (Figure 6–4).

Notice that the prevalence of breast cancer in these two groups, which is the same as the average pretest

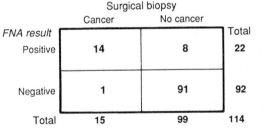

**Figure 6–4.** Comparison of FNA test results with findings from surgical excisional biopsies in women without palpable breast masses and in women with palpable breast masses. (Data on women without palpable breast masses reproduced, with permission, from Smith C et al: Fine-needle aspiration cytology in the diagnosis of primary breast cancer. Surgery 1988;103:178. Data on women with palpable breast masses reproduced, with permission, from, Bibbo M et al: Stereotaxic fine needle aspiration cytology of clinically occult malignant and premalignant breast lesions. Acta Cytol 1988;32:193.)

probability of disease for individual patients in the corresponding groups, was higher among the women with palpable masses (38%) than among the women without palpable masses (13%). Although the FNA test had identical specificity and sensitivity in these two clinical situations, the PV$^+$ of the test was 64% for women without palpable masses but 88% for women with palpable masses. *The PV$^+$ increased as the pretest probability of disease increased.* Therefore, it was easier to confirm the presence of breast cancer in a women with increased baseline likelihood of disease.

The PV$^-$ was 99% when the FNA test was used among women without palpable masses but decreased to 96% when used for women with palpable masses. The PV$^-$ decreased as the pretest probability of disease increased, as logically it should, since a disease is easier to exclude, the lower the probability of disease before the test is performed. The differences in predictive value between these two populations is due only to the difference in the pretest probability of disease, based upon whether a palpable mass was present.

Does the difference in predictive values described in Figure 6–4 have clinical implications? As discussed previously, among women with nonpalpable lesions, a negative FNA test (PV$^-$ = 99%) could reduce the probability of disease to 1%, and therefore obviate the need for a surgical biopsy. In the group with palpable masses, after a negative FNA test, the probability of breast cancer still would be 4%, which might warrant further testing such as biopsy. If neither a positive nor a negative test result would change subsequent management, one would question the use of the FNA test among women with palpable lumps.

## CUTOFF POINTS

In this chapter the use of the FNA test was analyzed as a detection method for breast cancer, assuming that the report of the FNA test would read either "cancer present" or "cancer absent." The dichotomous classification of clinical findings as positive or negative is commonplace and useful. Examples of dichotomous results are a positive or negative history of pain in a breast, the presence or absence of a palpable breast mass on physical examination, and a normal or abnormal alkaline phosphatase level (a serum marker of metastatic spread of breast cancer to bones or liver).

In reality, however, test results often occur along a continuum and do not have just positive or negative outcomes. A history of breast pain can be negative, intermittent, or continuous. The size of a breast mass may be measured in centimeters. A serum alkaline phosphatase level may range along a continuous

scale. In general, the more extreme the value of a continuous test result, the more likely that it reflects either a laboratory error or an abnormality in the patient.

The results of the FNA test often are classified as follows: (1) insufficient material to adequately assess presence or absence of malignancy; (2) benign (no malignant cells present); (3) suspicious (atypical cells present, but not definitely malignant); and (4) malignant cells present.

The choice of whether to consider each of the four possible results above as positive or negative influences the assessment of test performance. In both of the clinical series of patients with breast abnormalities presented above (see Figure 6–4), the patients with inadequate specimens were considered to have negative test results. Another important decision concerning the FNA test is whether or not to classify those women with suspicious or atypical results as positive or negative. The ramifications of this decision were explored in an evaluation of the FNA test among women with palpable breast masses. The evaluation of the FNA test is shown in Figure 6–5 using two different assumptions: (1) suspicious FNA tests were considered to be positive, and (2) suspicious FNA tests were considered to be negative. Note that the sensitivity of the FNA decreased and the specificity increased when women with suspicious FNAs were considered to have negative test results.

This is an example of changing the **cutoff point,** which is the point at which one considers the test to change from negative to positive. In Figure 6–5 where suspicious FNA results were thought to be positive, the cutoff point was considered to be between normal FNAs and suspicious FNAs. Where suspicious FNA results were considered to be negative, a cutoff point between a suspicious FNA and a malignant FNA was chosen. Moving the cutoff point changes the test's sensitivity, specificity, positive and negative predictive values, and hence, the way in which the test is used.

As illustrated in Figure 6–5, a negative FNA test result would reduce the probability of breast cancer, but with 4% chance of breast cancer might still warrant a biopsy. A positive FNA test result would increase the likelihood of cancer to 88%, but still would not absolutely confirm the diagnosis. Alternatively, by setting the cutoff point between the suspicious and malignant categories, the positive PV of the test becomes 100%. This could be useful clinically, since women with a positive FNA would require no further diagnostic tests prior to definitive surgical treatment (usually partial or complete removal of the affected breast). Indeed, the positive FNA has been characterized by many clinicians as a test that precludes the need for surgical excisional biopsy, thereby saving the patient an additional procedure and reducing the costs of treatment.

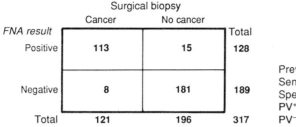

**Suspicious FNA results considered positive**

Surgical biopsy

| FNA result | Cancer | No cancer | Total |
|---|---|---|---|
| Positive | 113 | 15 | 128 |
| Negative | 8 | 181 | 189 |
| Total | 121 | 196 | 317 |

Prevalence = 38%
Sensitivity = 93%
Specificity = 92%
PV+ = 88%
PV− = 96%

**Suspicious FNA results considered negative**

Surgical biopsy

| FNA result | Cancer | No cancer | Total |
|---|---|---|---|
| Positive | 91 | 0 | 91 |
| Negative | 30 | 196 | 226 |
| Total | 121 | 196 | 317 |

Prevalence = 38%
Sensitivity = 75%
Specificity = 100%
PV+ = 100%
PV− = 87%

**Figure 6–5.** Comparison of FNA test results with findings from surgical excisional biopsies among women with palpable breast masses. (Data reproduced, with permission, from Bibbo M et al: Stereotaxic fine needle aspiration cytology of clinically occult and premalignant breast lesions. Acta Cytol 1988;32:193.)

## SCREENING TESTS

In the Patient Profile, a mammogram was recommended to the patient as a **screening test** for breast cancer. The purpose of the mammogram was to detect breast cancer earlier in the course of the disease than would occur if the test were not performed. Figure 6–6 is a schematic representation of the course of disease over time, and illustrates the possibility of detecting disease earlier using a screening test, thereby allowing for more effective treatment and prolonged survival. Inherent in this schematic diagram are two important concepts: (1) persons with a disease can be identified by use of a screening test before the time of routine diagnosis (eg, when symptoms occur), and (2) treatment at the time of detection by screening, as opposed to the time of routine diagnosis, results in an improved chance of survival.

Breast cancer is a prototypical example of a progressive disease. As with most malignancies, a breast cancer is believed to begin as a single malignant cell, which grows rapidly and forms a growing tumor mass. Over time, breast cancer cells can spread through the lymphatic system to the axillary lymph nodes and eventually to other parts of the body via the lymphatic system, the vascular system, or both. The earlier in the course of the disease that breast cancer is discovered, the less likely that the cancer will spread to lymph nodes and other sites.

It has been known for many years that length of survival from time of diagnosis of breast cancer is related to the size of the tumor and amount of spread of the breast cancer. When mammography was first introduced, it was obvious that cancerous lesions in the breast that could not be felt by even the most skilled clinician could be detected. Researchers pos-

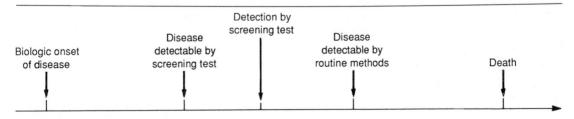

**Figure 6–6.** The natural history of a disease over time, including the preclinical stage at which the disease can be detected by a screening test.

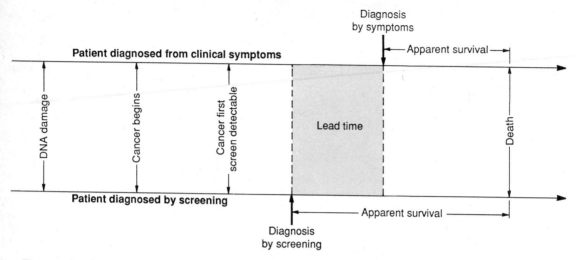

**Figure 6–7.** A comparison of a patient with a routine clinical diagnosis of disease and a patient with disease detected by screening. The shaded area represents the lead time between detection by screening and routine diagnosis.

tulated that by screening asymptomatic women with mammography, breast cancer could be detected at an earlier stage in the disease process, and affected women, therefore, would experience increased survival. This logic seems infallible, but two important biases—**lead-time bias** and **length-biased sampling**—must be considered when considering any screening program.

Lead-time bias is illustrated in Figure 6–7. *Lead-time bias is an increase in survival as measured from disease detection until death, without lengthening of life.* Notice in Figure 6–7 that the person detected with screening and the person detected without screening die at the exact same time, but the time from diagnosis until death is greater for the screened patient because the cancer was recognized earlier. The time from early diagnosis by screening to routine diagnosis is defined as the lead time.

*Length-biased sampling occurs when disease detected by a screening program is less aggressive than disease detected without screening.* On average, breast cancers detected in a screening program may be less aggressive than cancers that are diagnosed when symptoms appear. This occurs because less aggressive cancers typically grow more slowly than more aggressive cancers, and therefore the length of time that a cancer is detectable by screening is greater for slow-growing cancers. If one was to measure length of survival, the individuals with breast cancers detected by screening would appear to live longer because the cancers in these patients grow more slowly than the cancers in routinely diagnosed patients.

To overcome lead-time bias and length-biased sampling, and therefore assess the true benefit of a screening program, it is useful to measure disease-specific mortality rates within an entire population. Individuals who are either randomly assigned to a screening program or who receive no screening are followed to determine mortality from the disease of interest. Such a study was performed in the 1960s by the Health Insurance Plan (HIP) of New York. In the HIP study, women were randomly assigned to receive routine care or a screening program comprised of yearly mammographic and breast examinations.

The results of the study concerning the usefulness of mammography as a screening tool are presented in Figure 6–8. An issue in the evaluation of a screening test is to identify the false-negative tests. In the HIP study, asymptomatic women in the screened group with a positive screening test were referred for biopsy. There was no "gold-standard" test in this situation, ie, there was no existing definitive test, such as the FNA test, that could be performed among healthy women after the mammogram to determine whether cancers had been missed with screening. An approximation of the number of false-negative screening tests (47 in this example) was derived by determining the number of cancers that arose between yearly screening examinations; these were designated "interval" cancers. If a symptomatic cancer occurred after a screening mammogram, but prior to the next mammogram, the first mammogram was presumed to have been falsely negative.

In Figure 6–8, notice that mammography had an excellent specificity (98%), yet the false-positive tests still outnumbered the true-positive tests by over 7 to 1 (PV$^+$ = 12%). This means that among women with positive mammograms who were referred for a definitive diagnosis as a result of surgical biopsy, more than seven biopsies were negative for every breast cancer that was found. This high false-positive rate is

Disease status

|  | Cancer | No cancer | Total |
|---|---|---|---|
| Mammography<br>Positive | 132 | 985 | 1,117 |
| Negative | 47 | 62,295 | 62,342 |
| Total | 179 | 63,280 | 63,459 |

Prevalence = 0.3%
Sensitivity = 73.7%
Specificity = 98.4%
PV⁺ = 11.8%
PV⁻ = 99.9%

**Figure 6–8.** Results of mammographic screening in the Health Insurance Plan (HIP) of New York study. (Data reproduced, with permission, from Shapiro S et al: *Periodic Screening for Breast Cancer: The Health Insurance Plan Project and its Sequelae, 1963–1986.* Johns Hopkins, 1988.)

related to the low prevalence of breast cancer in the general population. A low PV⁺ is fairly typical for a screening test that is used to detect a disease that is relatively infrequent in the general population at any point in time. It is important, therefore, to consider the possible anxiety, expense, and morbidity associated with false-positive results when screening initiatives are introduced into the general population.

The purpose of the HIP study was to determine if repeated use of mammography reduced breast cancer mortality. The use of a concurrent control group allowed an assessment of the relationship between being offered mammographic screening and mortality from breast cancer. A random assignment of women to either screening or routine care tended to balance the screened and unscreened groups with respect to factors that might affect subsequent breast cancer mortality (see discussion of randomization in Chapter 7). Evaluation of age-specific breast cancer mortality rates rather than length of survival diminished the possible distorting effect of lead-time bias. After the initial screening, slowly growing tumors presumably were removed from the screened women, and the effectiveness of subsequent annual mammograms in reducing breast cancer mortality was less likely to reflect length-biased sampling. At the conclusion of the study, the researchers concluded that mammography reduced breast cancer mortality among the screened population by 30% when compared to the control group of women receiving routine care. The results of this landmark study, combined with findings from investigations of similar design in other countries, established the effectiveness of mammographic screening.

A list of criteria for a successful screening program is presented in Table 6–1. A mammographic screening program for breast cancer can be assessed using these criteria. Breast cancer is an important public health problem in the United States; one out of every nine women will be diagnosed with breast cancer at some time during her lifetime. Early detection of breast cancer allows less extensive surgical treatment and reduces morbidity and mortality from this disease. Since breast cancer incidence increases steadily

with age, a high-risk population can be defined as any group of women who are over 50 years of age. Many experts recommend that women between ages 40 and 49 have a mammogram every 2 years and that women aged 50 or older have a mammogram once a year. Although the test does cause some discomfort, most women find the procedure acceptable. There is an extremely small risk of breast cancer associated with the radiation received during mammography. This increased risk is negligible when compared to an average woman's baseline risk of the disease, however. Finally, mammography is a relatively sensitive and specific test.

## SUMMARY

In this chapter, the principles of evaluating and interpreting diagnostic tests were introduced, using the diagnosis of breast cancer as an example. The process of reaching a diagnosis can be represented as a weighing of probabilities. When a particular diagnosis is excluded or ruled out, then the probability of that disease is close to 0. When a particular diagnosis is confirmed, then the probability of that disease is close to 100%. The challenge for the clinician is to collect information that will allow successive improvements in probability until a disease is either confirmed or excluded.

All clinical information is subject to error. Ac-

**Table 6–1.** Criteria for a successful screening program.

Morbidity or mortality of the disease must be a sufficient concern to public health.
Effective early intervention must be known to reduce morbidity or mortality.
A high-risk population must exist.
The screening test should be sensitive and specific.
The screening test must be acceptable to the target population.
Minimal risk should be associated with the screening test.
Diagnostic workup for a positive test result must have acceptable morbidity given the number of false-positive results.

counting for the various errors that can arise in diagnostic testing allows the physician to select tests and interpret the results of these tests appropriately. One type of error is referred to as **false-negative,** because the test fails to detect a disease when it is present. A test is said to be **sensitive** when the percentage of false-negative errors is low. A second type of error is referred to as **false-positive,** because the test indicates that a disease is present when in fact it is not. A test with a low percentage of false-positive results is said to be **specific.**

Sensitivity and specificity are characteristics of a diagnostic test. It is useful to consider two other measures, **positive predictive value** (PV $^+$) and **negative predictive value** (PV $^-$), which are used to interpret the results of a diagnostic test. PV $^+$ is the percentage of persons with positive test results who truly have the disease of interest. PV $^-$ is the percentage of persons with negative test results who actually do not have the disease of interest. Both positive and negative predictive values are heavily influenced by either the pretest probability that the patient has the disease of interest, or, in the population setting, by the prevalence of the disease in the particular population that is tested.

In some situations, a test result has only one of two possible outcomes: positive or negative. In other circumstances, however, multiple levels or even a continuous range of values can occur. For multilevel or continuous outcome test results, a dividing line or **cutoff point** can be chosen to separate findings considered to be positive or negative. The choice of a cutoff value will affect the sensitivity and specificity of a test, and consequently the positive and negative predictive values as well. Raising the threshold for considering a result to be positive typically will be accompanied by a gain in specificity (fewer false-positives) but a loss of sensitivity (more false-negatives or missed cases). On the other hand, lowering the threshold for considering a result to be positive typically will reduce the level of false-negatives (raise sensitivity) and increase the likelihood of false-positives (lower specificity).

The use of tests to detect a disease at an earlier time than it would be diagnosed through routine methods is referred to as **screening.** The evaluation of a screening test must take into account two types of distorting effects: **lead-time bias** and **length-biased sampling.** Lead-time bias can occur in a comparison of survival time, since cases detected by screening are known to have the disease earlier in the clinical course and therefore may appear to survive longer even if the time of death is the same had no screening occurred. Lead-time bias may be minimized by evaluating mortality rates rather than duration of survival, as the outcome. Length-biased sampling can occur when the screening test preferentially detects slowly progressive disease that is less likely to cause death or may result in a delayed death. Length-biased sampling can be reduced by repeated screening efforts, since the slowly progressive forms of disease are likely to be removed by the initial screening and should not be overrepresented in later screenings.

A successful screening program requires focus on a disease with considerable morbidity and mortality that can be diagnosed and treated effectively at an early stage. In addition, the ability to define a high-risk population to whom the test can be acceptably administered with minimal risk is essential. The false-negative, and particularly the false-positive, errors of the screening test should be relatively small, and the expense and morbidity of further evaluation of false positives must be acceptable. When evaluated using these criteria, screening mammography is judged to be a very useful technique.

## STUDY QUESTIONS

**Directions:** For each question, select the single best answer.

**Questions 1–5:** A comparison of clinically diagnosed versus autopsy confirmed myocardial infarctions was performed among 1000 consecutive deceased patients, as shown in Figure 6–9.

1. From these data, the prevalence of myocardial infarction at autopsy was closest to:
    A. 20%
    B. 67%
    C. 80%
    D. 90%
    E. 95%

2. The sensitivity of the clinical diagnosis was closest to:
    A. 20%
    B. 67%
    C. 80%
    D. 90%
    E. 95%

3. The specificity of the clinical diagnosis was closest to:
    A. 20%
    B. 67%

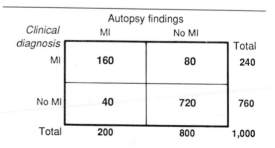

| Clinical diagnosis | Autopsy findings | | Total |
|---|---|---|---|
| | MI | No MI | |
| MI | 160 | 80 | 240 |
| No MI | 40 | 720 | 760 |
| Total | 200 | 800 | 1,000 |

**Figure 6–9.** Comparison of clinical diagnosis of myocardial infarction (MI) with autopsy findings in 1000 consecutive patients who underwent autopsy.

**C.** 80%
**D.** 90%
**E.** 95%

**4.** The positive predictive value of a clinical diagnosis was closest to:
**A.** 20%
**B.** 67%
**C.** 80%
**D.** 80%
**E.** 95%

**5.** The negative predictive value of a clinical diagnosis was closest to:
**A.** 20%
**B.** 67%
**C.** 80%
**D.** 90%
**E.** 95%

**Questions 6–10:** A comparison of clinically diagnosed versus autopsy-confirmed gastric and peptic ulcers was performed in 10,000 consecutive deceased patients, as shown in Figure 6–10.

**6.** From these data, the prevalence of autopsy-confirmed gastric and peptic ulcer was closest to:
**A.** 3%
**B.** 43%
**C.** 87%
**D.** 98%
**E.** 100%

**7.** The sensitivity of a clinical diagnosis was closest to:
**A.** 3%
**B.** 43%
**C.** 87%
**D.** 98%
**E.** 100%

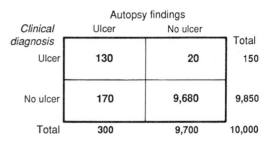

| Clinical | Autopsy findings | | |
|---|---|---|---|
| diagnosis | Ulcer | No ulcer | Total |
| Ulcer | 130 | 20 | 150 |
| No ulcer | 170 | 9,680 | 9,850 |
| Total | 300 | 9,700 | 10,000 |

**Figure 6–10.** Comparison of clinical diagnosis of gastric and peptic ulcer with autopsy findings in 10,000 consecutive patients who underwent autopsy.

**8.** The specificity of a clinical diagnosis was closest to:
**A.** 3%
**B.** 43%
**C.** 87%
**D.** 98%
**E.** 100%

**9.** The positive predictive value of a clinical diagnosis was closest to:
**A.** 3%
**B.** 43%
**C.** 87%
**D.** 98%
**E.** 100%

**10.** The negative predictive value of a clinical diagnosis was closest to:
**A.** 3%
**B.** 43%
**C.** 87%
**D.** 98%
**E.** 100%

**FURTHER READING**

Anderson RE, Hill RB, Key CR: The sensitivity and specificity of clinical diagnostics during five decades. JAMA 1989;261:1610.

**REFERENCES**

Bibbo M et al: Stereotaxic fine needle aspiration cytology of clinically occult malignant and premalignant breast lesions. Acta Cytol 1988;32:193.

Osler W: Medical education. In: *Counsels and Ideals,* 2nd ed. Houghton Mifflin, 1921.

Shapiro S et al: Breast cancers detected–sensitivity and specificity of screening. In: *Periodic Screening For Breast Cancer: The Health Insurance Plan Project and Its Sequelae, 1963–1986.* Johns Hopkins, 1988.

Smith C et al: Fine-needle aspiration cytology in the diagnosis of primary breast cancer. Surgery 1988;103:178.

# 7

# Clinical Trials

## PATIENT PROFILE

*A 56-year-old automobile mechanic called his family physician at 6 AM complaining of being awakened by crushing pain in the middle of his chest. The pain had not changed in intensity since onset 15 minutes before the call. The patient also reported sweating, nausea, and a sharp pain shooting down his left arm to the elbow. The physician advised the patient to call an ambulance for transportation to the hospital emergency room, where a more thorough evaluation could be performed.*

*In the emergency room, the physician obtained a more complete history and determined that the patient had experienced similar but less intense pain for the past week when performing strenuous work but that the pain had always resolved with rest. Physical examination was normal except for a slightly elevated pulse rate of 100 beats/min and the presence of diaphoresis. Chest x-ray was normal, but an electrocardiogram showed signs of anterior myocardial ischemia.*

*Based on the history, physical examination, and ECG, the diagnosis of acute myocardial infarction was made, and the physician formulated a treatment plan. The patient was moved to the intensive care unit and therapy was initiated.*

## CLINICAL BACKGROUND

Twenty years ago, the treatment plan for a patient with myocardial infarction may have consisted of rest plus morphine and nitroglycerin (to decrease pain and increase blood flow to the ischemic myocardium). Today, however, a number of additional different treatment plans would be considered, including surgically bypassing the atherosclerotic coronary artery lesions, dilating the constricted coronary arteries with a radiographically directed balloon, or lysing blood clots in the coronary arteries with medications.

The ability to lyse blood clots by pharmacologic means is among the newest and most promising treatments for myocardial infarction. Drugs such as streptokinase, urokinase, and alteplase (tissue plasminogen

activator; tPA) can be infused through a peripheral vein or directly into the coronary arteries in order to lyse clots within the arteries (Figure 7–1). The use of these thrombolytic agents within the first 4 hours after a heart attack can reduce myocardial tissue damage and increase survival rates among heart attack patients.

In theory, tPA has two advantages over streptokinase. First, streptokinase is not a human-derived protein and for that reason is more likely to cause serious allergic responses than tPA, which is a human-derived factor. Second and more importantly, tPA is thought to be active only at a site of thrombosis, whereas streptokinase induces a systemic "lytic state." Therefore, it is hoped that tPA may be as effective as streptokinase (or more so) without increasing a patient's risk of experiencing the most severe complication of lytic therapy—bleeding. tPA, however, is much more expensive than streptokinase. While a theoretic advantage would tend to favor the use of tPA, it would be useful to perform a study to compare these two treatments. *A randomized controlled clinical trial is a study design in which one treatment is compared directly with another treatment to determine which of the two options would be of greatest benefit.*

## INTRODUCTION TO CLINICAL TRIALS

In the Patient Profile, the clinician is faced with a treatment decision: whether to use streptokinase or tPA. Hippocrates' axiom—"First, do no harm"—is a time-honored warning to clinicians contemplating medical intervention. "One must attend in medical practice not primarily to plausible theories," Hippocrates wrote, "but to experience combined with reason." In other words, a treatment plan should seem reasonable in theory but should also be tested experientially. Over 2000 years ago, Hippocrates noted the importance of actual patients' receiving a treatment in judging that treatment's benefits.

In modern medical practice, a randomized, controlled clinical trial of one therapy versus another is the accepted standard by which the usefulness of a

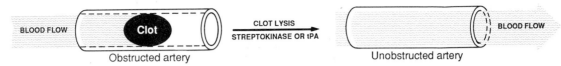

**Figure 7–1.** Schematic representation of clot lysis therapy for removing blockages of the coronary arteries.

treatment is judged. To practice modern medicine and select appropriate therapy, one must understand the design and conduct of clinical trials.

This important method of evaluating treatments utilizes two types of knowledge, both alluded to by Hippocrates: reason and experience. "Reasonable" treatment is that which is suggested by a knowledge of the basic sciences of medicine. For the clinical situation presented in the Patient Profile, a knowledge of the pathophysiology of coronary heart disease, the mechanism of clot formation and lysis, and the pharmacologic effects of tPA and streptokinase would favor the use of tPA, since that drug should lead to lysis of clots in the coronary arteries while exposing the patient to a lesser risk of dangerous side effects. As stated by Hippocrates, however, the clinician cannot base therapeutic decisions on theory alone but must submit the dictates of reason to the test of experience and react appropriately.

Clinicians employ two types of experience when assessing a treatment regimen—their own personal experience and the written or orally conveyed experience of their colleagues. Written experience may take the form of a report of a single case, a series of cases, or a comparison of one treatment versus another. *The direct comparison of two or more treatment modalities in human groups is referred to as a "clinical trial."* The development of the clinical trial is a product of the application of modern scientific method to clinical medicine. The purpose of the clinical trial is to provide clinicians with information that will help them prescribe appropriate, timely treatment for their patients.

Experiments on human populations have inherent difficulties not found in the laboratory. The laboratory scientist can carefully control the conditions under which an experiment is conducted. For instance, genetically identical male mice 30 days old may be divided into two groups, kept in the same environment, and given identical diets except for a single micronutrient to ascertain the effect of that nutrient on the development of disease. Human beings, however—except for the rare exception of identical twins—are variable in their genetic make-ups as well as their environments. Control of a human subject's environment or compliance with a treatment regimen cannot be controlled, as it can in conducting animal experiments. Furthermore, human patients and researchers have direct personal interests in the outcomes of trials. To acknowledge and account for the

complexities of the human subject is the challenge of conducting a clinical trial.

## STATEMENT OF THE RESEARCH QUESTIONS

The first step in performing a clinical trial—as in a laboratory experiment as well—is to formulate the major research question. This question usually is referred to as a hypothesis and is refined to determine important study parameters, such as the types of interventions to be compared, the nature of the outcomes to be assessed, the number of subjects in each treatment group, and the eligibility requirements for enrollment.

The parameter that is measured to answer the most important question of the clinical trial is the **primary end point.** When determining the primary end point, clinical researchers must consider the following questions:

**(1)** Which end points are the most clinically important?

**(2)** Which of these end points can be measured in a reasonable manner?

**(3)** What practical constraints exist, such as population size, financial resources of the research study, and ability to follow patients on a long-term basis?

Researchers in Australia designed a clinical trial to address the following question: *Is streptokinase or tPA "superior" in the treatment of patients with acute myocardial infarction?*

More than one end point can be measured to assess treatment efficacy. Types of end points include measures of quality of life, length of survival, percentage of patients surviving, complication rate, and intermediate end points which are predictive of survival or quality of life (Table 7–1). In assessing "superiority" for treatment of myocardial infarction, possible outcome measures include the percentage of patients surviving for at least 1 month following treatment; a patient's ability to exercise or return to work; the risk of having a major complication from treatment; the risk of experiencing congestive heart failure after infarction; the risk of having persistently clotted arteries after thrombolytic therapy; or a measure of left ventricular function, such as left ventricular ejection frac-

**Table 7–1.** Types and examples of end points used in clinical trials.

| Type of End Point | Example |
|---|---|
| Quality of life | Ability to perform usual daily tasks |
| Survival | Percentage of patients alive 1 year after entering trial |
| Complications | Percentage of patients who develop serious allergic reactions |
| Intermediate measures | Percentage of patients who have recurrence of symptoms |

tion (LVEF)—the percentage of blood ejected by the left ventricle during systolic contraction. Examples of two of these questions restated symbolically as hypotheses follow:

$$H_0 : \pi_0 = \pi_1$$

where $H_0$ is the so-called **null hypothesis** and $\pi_0$ and $\pi_1$ are the percentages of persons surviving to 1 year following treatment in the streptokinase and tPA groups, respectively.

$$H_0 : \mu_0 = \mu_1$$

where $\mu_0$ and $\mu_1$ are the mean LVEFs for persons in the streptokinase and tPA groups, respectively.

Note that these hypotheses are stated in the null form—ie, *there is no difference between the treatment groups regarding the specified end point.* The purpose of the clinical trial is to test whether the observed outcomes are consistent with these null hypotheses. If the observed data are not consistent with the null hypothesis, then the null hypothesis ($H_0$) is rejected in favor of an **alternative hypothesis** ($H_A$) such as the following:

$$H_A : \pi_0 \neq \pi_1$$

where $\pi_0$ and $\pi_1$ again are the respective percentages of survivors at 1 year following treatment in the streptokinase and tPA groups. This alternative hypothesis states that the two treatments will differ with respect to 1-year survival. Similarly, an alternative hypothesis for the LVEF outcome could be stated as follows:

$$H_A : \mu_0 \neq \mu_1$$

where $\mu_0$ and $\mu_1$ again are the respective mean LVEFs for the streptokinase and tPA groups. In other words, this alternative hypothesis states that the two treatments will differ with respect to mean LVEF achieved in patients after treatment.

Regarding the streptokinase-tPA question, important clinical end points include 1-year survival and quality of life after survival, but the researchers chose to study LVEF as the primary end point of the study. The researchers chose this particular end point for several reasons:

**(1)** LVEF is a quantitative measure of cardiac function that is easily understood and commonly used as a predictor of the extent of myocardial infarction as well as of heart failure and death after infarction.
**(2)** LVEF can be measured in a timely manner postinfarction, circumventing the need for long-term follow-up of patients, which can be both difficult and costly.
**(3)** The researchers knew that they would not be able to enter enough subjects in the trial— given the expense and their population of patients—to adequately answer questions concerning 1-year survival.

LVEF is an "intermediate" end point, which is thought to be predictive of two important final end points: survival and quality of life. LVEF, therefore, was chosen as the primary end point in this study for three reasons: (1) because it was thought to be a predictor of important clinical end points; (2) because it could be easily and inexpensively measured; and (3) because an adequate sample size was available to make the study of posttreatment differences in LVEF feasible.

## SAMPLE SIZE DETERMINATION

The number of subjects who should be enrolled in a clinical trial—ie, the sample size—must be determined at the same time as the primary research end point. At the conclusion of any experiment, data are analyzed and a statistical decision is made to either accept or reject the study hypothesis. This decision is based upon probabilities and, unfortunately, may be correct or incorrect. The relationship between the possible results of the streptokinase-tPA trial and the "truth" is shown in Figure 7–2. For the purposes of this discussion, "truth" can be thought of as the results of the intervention if applied correctly to the entire universe of patients with the clinical condition under study. A clinical trial can be thought of as a sample of the "truth." Using a sample of the entire population, one hopes to make valid inferences about the entire population, but since one can intervene on only a sample, there are risks of arriving at mistaken conclusions.

In cells A and D of Figure 7–2, the results of the study agree with the "truth." In cells B and C, however, the study results do not agree with the "truth"—

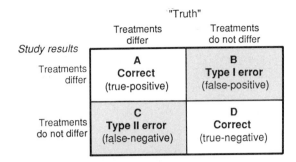

**Figure 7–2.** Comparison of study results and "truth."

ie, errors are made. These two types of error differ in their origin and implications.

*If the study finds a difference in treatments, when in actuality there is no difference (cell B), then a type I error is present.* Under this circumstance, the *study results are falsely positive.* In the streptokinase-tPA example, a type I error would occur if the investigators concluded that there was a difference between treatments in the mean LVEF achieved, when in "truth" there was no difference in mean LVEF. *If the study fails to find a difference in treatments when in actuality there is a difference (cell C), a type II error is said to have occurred.* Under this circumstance, *the study results are falsely negative.* In the streptokinase-tPA trial, a type II error would occur if the investigators concluded that there was no difference between treatments in the mean LVEF achieved when in "truth" one of the treatments produced a superior mean LVEF.

Falsely positive or falsely negative studies can occur because of faulty methodology, because of chance occurrences, or for both reasons. While methodologic error can be minimized by careful attention to study design, errors due to chance can never be completely eliminated. Such errors, however, can be estimated. The notation used to denote the likelihood of a type I error—that the difference observed between groups is not a true difference but due instead to chance— is the **alpha level.** Conversely, the notation used to describe the likelihood of a type II error—that the study did not find a difference when there indeed is a difference—is called the **beta level.** Researchers specify the alpha and beta levels when planning a study. The alpha level is specified commonly as 0.05, which means that the investigator is willing to accept a 5% risk of committing a type I error (falsely concluding that the groups differ when in reality they do not). The investigator must also specify beforehand the beta level, or risk of committing a type II error. Often a level of 0.20 for beta is considered adequate—in other words, a one in five chance of missing a true difference between the groups is allowed. The **statistical power,** or ability of a study to detect a true difference between groups, is $(1 - \beta)$.

Statistical power for a study with a beta level of 0.20 would be 0.80, or 80%. Such a study would have an 80% chance of detecting a specified difference in outcome between the treatment groups.

Once the alpha and beta levels have been specified, the research team must specify another extremely important study parameter before determining sample size—the magnitude of the difference in outcome between treatment groups that the study will be designed to detect. This difference between the treatments under comparison is of great importance and should be selected on the basis of clinical information. In deciding on the level of outcome difference worthy of detection, the investigator might consider one or more of the following questions:

**(1)** What difference in outcome would be important to clinicians treating this type of patient?
**(2)** What difference would be meaningful to a patient who may suffer the consequences of the disease?
**(3)** What difference in outcome would justify use of the more effective treatment in spite of greater expense or greater side effects?

Formulas for the determination of sample size and illustrative calculations are provided in Appendix B. Suffice it to say here that all three factors just mentioned (acceptable levels of type I and type II errors and the expected magnitude of difference in outcome between groups) are inversely related to the required sample size (Table 7–2). That is, if one can tolerate only a 1% chance of committing a type I error rather than accepting a 5% error level, then the sample size must be increased. Similarly, a decrease in the acceptable level of type II error (enhanced statistical power) is accompanied by a need to study more subjects.

As the expected magnitude of difference in outcome (eg, mean LVEF) between treatment groups decreases, a larger sample size is required to detect the difference. In contrast, as the variability of the outcome (eg, the standard deviation of LVEF) diminishes, fewer subjects are required to demonstrate a difference in outcome between the groups.

**Table 7–2.** Factors that affect sample size requirements.

| Factor | Effect on Sample Size Required |
|---|---|
| ↓ Acceptable type I error | ↑ |
| ↓ Acceptable type II error | ↑ |
| ↓ Variability of outcome measures | ↓ |
| ↓ Expected differences in outcome and between groups | ↑ |

## RANDOMIZATION

The central tenet of the clinical trial is that patients should be assigned to treatment groups by a method that maximizes the probability of the two groups' being similar in those background characteristics that may influence either the response to therapy or the primary outcome measure. For the modern clinical trial, the assignment to treatments is done by **randomization.** *With randomization, the determination of treatment group assignment is based upon probability alone and is not influenced by the physician's or patient's preference.*

The assignment for each patient is independent of the assignment for all other patients. That is to say, the treatment assignment of each patient is not influenced by the assignment of any other patient. When there are two possible treatment assignments with equal sample sizes (as in the streptokinase-tPA example), then every patient has a 50% chance of being assigned to either one of the treatments. Such an assignment could be decided by a coin toss: If the coin comes up heads, the patient is assigned to streptokinase; if the coin comes up tails, the patient is assigned to tPA. Of course, tossing a coin is a rather inelegant way to assign patients to treatment groups, so many investigators use more sophisticated devices, such as tables of random numbers or computer-generated random assignments. The basic design of a randomized controlled clinical trial is illustrated in Figure 7–3 using the streptokinase-tPA study as an example.

As recently as 50 years ago, the primary means of evaluating the benefit of a new treatment was to treat a series of patients with the new method and then compare the outcome with that observed in the past for a group of patients who received the standard therapy. The patients who received the standard therapy are called **nonconcurrent** or **historical controls.** Consider how such a study might have been performed to address the streptokinase-tPA question. If researchers wanted to test the hypothesis concerning the clinical efficacy of tPA (experimental treatment) versus streptokinase (standard or control treatment), a group of patients would be given tPA and the postinfarction mean LVEF of the tPA group would then be compared with the mean LVEF of a group of patients treated at an earlier time with streptokinase (Figure 7–4). There are several inherent problems with this approach:

(1) The diagnostic criteria for a myocardial infarction—or the technology available to diagnose a myocardial infarction—may change over time.
(2) The techniques used to measure LVEF may change over the time period of the study.
(3) Additional treatment modalities, such as more aggressive prehospital care, could become available over time and for ethical reasons would have to be employed on the patients during the second part of the study.
(4) Most importantly, the patients who presented with myocardial infarction during the time when patients were being treated with streptokinase may not have been similar in prognostic characteristics (sex, age, location of infarction) to the group who present during the tPA treatment period.

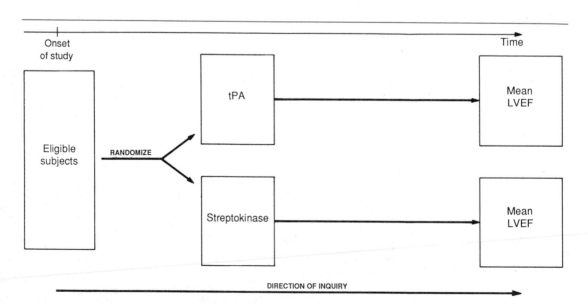

**Figure 7–3.** Schematic diagram of the design of a randomized controlled clinical trial comparing streptokinase with tPA for treatment of an initial myocardial infarction. LVEF = left ventricular ejection fraction.

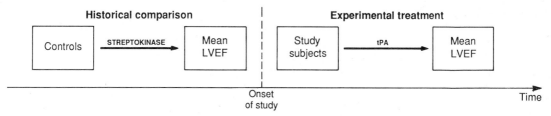

**Figure 7–4.** Schematic diagram of the comparison of tPA treatment for myocardial infarction against the historical experience of streptokinase treatment for previous patients with myocardial infarction. LVEF = left ventricular ejection fraction.

If concurrent controls are necessary to compare treatment groups, a basic question arises: *How should patients be assigned to each treatment group?*

One could have physicians or patients choose which treatment a patient will be given. This technique, however, is seriously flawed. Objective assessment of a patient's symptoms and signs is a requisite skill for any health care provider. Nevertheless, health care providers are empathic to the needs of their patients and often have opinions concerning the efficacy of a treatment prior to the results of clinical trials. Patients—who of course have a direct personal interest in any treatment result—would very likely choose a treatment based on their assessment or expectation of its efficacy.

In order to avoid unfair comparisons that may result from these preferences of patients and physicians, the assignment to treatment group should therefore be determined by chance, independently of the wishes of clinicians and patients. *The purpose of randomization is to achieve "equality" of baseline characteristics of treatment groups, so that the comparison of treatments is considered fair.* To assess the equality of the treatment groups, demographic and prognostic factors may be compared between groups. If patients indeed have been randomly allocated, it is expected that the groups will be similar in demographic and prognostic features. Table 7–3 is an example from the streptokinase-tPA trial of the comparison of treatment groups after randomization.

As can be seen in Table 7–3, these two treatment groups are remarkably similar with regard to sex, previous diseases, previous treatment with antihypertensives, systolic blood pressure, and pulse rate. There is a 4% difference between groups in the proportion of patients who had an anterior myocardial infarction (considered to be a more serious site of infarction). In order to control for this difference in treatment groups, the researchers analyzed separately the results of postinfarction LVEF for patients with anterior and inferior infarctions—ie, comparison of treatment effects was **stratified** by location of infarction during the analysis phase.

Stratification by important prognostic features can be performed during the randomization phase of the trial. If one wants to ensure that similar numbers of patients with certain important prognostic characteristics are included in each treatment group, those characteristics can be accounted for in the randomization process. In the streptokinase-tPA trial, for instance, patients with anterior myocardial infarction could be allocated in equal numbers to each of the two treatments. Suppose, for example, that for every four persons with an anterior infarction, two persons are assigned to tPA and two to streptokinase. The order in which the two treatments are assigned to the four patients would be random, and at the end of the study there would be an equal number of patients with anterior myocardial infarction in each study group. Assignment of patients in this manner is termed **block randomization.** *The purpose of randomization in blocks of patients is to protect against imbalanced treatment assignment (due to "luck of the draw") with respect to prognostically important patient subgroups.*

**Table 7–3.** Percent distribution of baseline characteristics of patients enrolled in the streptokinase-tPA trial.[1]

| | Treatment Group | |
|---|---|---|
| Characteristic | Streptokinase | tPA |
| Gender (male) | 79 | 81 |
| Previous history | | |
| Hypertension | 26 | 22 |
| Diabetes | 10 | 10 |
| Claudication | 3 | 3 |
| Angina (in past 3 months) | 15 | 11 |
| Smoking | 56 | 55 |
| Previous therapy | | |
| Beta-blockers | 15 | 11 |
| Calcium channel blockers | 5 | 7 |
| Infarct location | | |
| Anterior | 32 | 36 |
| Interior | 68 | 64 |
| Admission status | | |
| Systolic blood pressure (mm Hg) | 133 ± 26[2] | 132 ± 27 |
| Heart rate (beats/min) | 71 ± 16[2] | 71 ± 17 |

[1] Adapted and reproduced, with permission, from White HD et al: Effect of intravenous streptokinase as compared with that of tissue plasminogen activator on left ventricular function after first myocardial infarction. N Engl J Med 1989;320:817.
[2] Plus-minus values are means ± SD.

## THE PLACEBO EFFECT AND BLINDING

In the year 1801, Haygarth reported the results of what may have been the first **placebo-controlled trial.** A popular treatment for many diseases at that time was to apply metal rods, known as Perkins tractors, to the body and thus relieve symptoms through a supposed electromagnetic influence of the metal. Haygarth treated five patients with imitation wooden tractors and found that four gained relief. The following day, he used the metal tractors on the same five patients and obtained identical results: relief in four of the five subjects. In describing the results of his experiment, Haygarth quoted James Lind, who is credited with performing the first clinical trial: "An important lesson in physic is here to be learnt, viz., the wonderful and powerful influence of the passions of the mind upon the state and disorders of the body. This is too often overlooked in the cure of diseases . . . ."

The influence of treatment of any kind on patients' perceptions of their illness cannot be forgotten when designing a clinical trial. This concept is of greatest importance when the outcome measure is subjective. The patient's desires may also influence decisions made by clinicians subsequent to the initial randomization in a clinical trial. An additional factor that could potentially lead to differential treatment of groups within a trial is the clinician's decision process during a clinical trial. For example, will a clinician who has certain beliefs concerning a treatment's efficacy be likely to discontinue a therapy believed to be inferior in favor of the alternative therapy?

To account for the placebo effect and to reduce the introduction of bias due to patients' and clinicians' conceptions, studies may be conducted in a **blinded** fashion. *"Blinding" means that the treatment assignment is not known to certain persons* (Table 7–4). In a **single-blinded study,** the treatment assignment is not known to the patients; in a **double-blinded study,** the treatment assignment is not known either to the patients or to their physicians. In a double-blinded study, the treatment assignment is only revealed to the patient and physician if there are serious or unexpected side effects or when the study is completed.

In the streptokinase-tPA trial, patients were given two intravenous infusions, one over 30 minutes and

one over 2 hours. One of the infusions contained an active drug and the other was saline solution. Neither the patients nor their physicians knew which of the two drugs any individual patient was receiving. Therefore, this study is considered to be double-blinded. To further reduce the chance of bias, the measurement of LVEF was performed by physicians who had no knowledge of the patient or the treatment group. This was done to eliminate the possibility of **observer bias.**

Although blinding of both the patients and the treating physicians is desirable, there are trials that cannot be conducted in a blinded fashion because the treatments are so obviously different that it is not feasible to keep the assignment secret. Examples are heart surgery compared with drug therapy for coronary atherosclerosis or chemotherapy compared with no treatment for patients with lung cancer. Whenever possible, however, blinding should be employed, since lack of blinding could influence perceptions of outcome and reduce the confidence in study results.

## ETHICAL ISSUES CONCERNING CLINICAL TRIALS

The investigator who contemplates entering a patient into a randomized clinical trial is faced with several ethical dilemmas. First, is the randomized clinical trial method ethically acceptable? One of the most important ethical tenets in medicine is that the patient's welfare is of primary concern, and a caregiver should prescribe the optimal treatment for a patient. One could argue that even if a clinician has only a "hunch" or "feeling" that one treatment is superior, the patient should be offered that treatment. Randomization between two treatments, therefore, might be considered to be unethical. Given the seriousness and possible side effects of medical interventions, however, the axiom "first, do no harm" must always be borne in mind. The history of medicine is replete with examples of treatments now known to be either of no benefit or actually harmful. The clinical trial is considered to be the best method available for determining the benefits and potential harm of treatment regimens.

If one accepts that the clinical trial method is acceptable, then one must decide how to perform trials as ethically as possible. What follows is a list of guidelines for medical professionals conducting clinical trials:

(1) None of the treatment options included in a randomized trial should be known to be inferior to another based on previous randomized studies, and if a standard treatment regimen exists, it should be used as the control.

(2) The trial should address a question that is of clini-

**Table 7–4.** Summary of various types of blinding to assignment of treatment in clinical trials.

| Blinding | Knowledge of Treatment Assignment | |
|---|---|---|
| | Patient | Investigator |
| None | Yes | Yes |
| Single | No | Yes |
| Double | No | No |

cal importance and seek to answer the question in a way that will be useful for future patients.

(3) Patients should be told that they are part of a clinical experiment and should be informed in understandable language about all treatment options, their risks and benefits, and the nature of randomization. The patient who then agrees to participate is said to have given **informed consent,** which implies that the patient freely chooses to be included in the trial.

(4) The investigators beginning the trial should be able to recruit the number of patients needed to meet the required sample size in a timely manner.

## EVALUATION OF CLINICAL TRIALS

Relatively few physicians design clinical trials, and a limited number enter patients into clinical trials—but all clinicians read published accounts of clinical trials and use the results to guide their treatment of patients. A checklist of questions to help the physician interpret and evaluate these trials is included as Table 7–5.

### Design Issues

The null hypothesis and what would constitute a meaningful difference in outcome should be stated in the methods section of a reported clinical trial. In the streptokinase-tPA trial, the primary outcome and the difference that was considered meaningful were clearly stated. Trials should be designed to test one specific hypothesis or only a few hypotheses, and these should be evident to the reader.

The characteristics of the study population are especially important when assessing the relevance of a particular trial to an individual practitioner's patients. In the streptokinase-tPA trial, the eligibility and exclusion criteria are clearly stated, as summarized in Table 7–6. Summary data about gender, age, and medical histories of the participants were shown previously in Table 7–3. The combination of the entry criteria and the demographic characteristics of the study entrants provides the reader with an adequate description of the study group. With this information, the reader is better able to judge whether the results of this study are applicable to a particular patient. Often, patients are excluded from a trial for pragmatic reasons, such as inability to comply with treatment or lack of fluency in the language of the investigators. These exclusions, however, may limit the ability to generalize study findings to other patient groups.

Once randomized to a particular treatment regimen, a patient may adhere to that regimen (comply) or may elect not to follow the prescribed regimen. Possible reasons for noncompliance are listed in Table 7–7. The investigator cannot force participants to comply, since such coercion would violate the rights of subjects to participate of their own free choice. There are several possible ways to increase com-

**Table 7–5.** Checklist for evaluating clinical trials.

1. What was the null hypothesis?
   a. What was the outcome of interest?
   b. What was thought to be a meaningful difference in outcome?
2. What group was being tested?
   a. How was the study population for the trial selected?
      (1) Exclusion criteria
      (2) Random versus volunteer
   b. What were the group's demographic and health characteristics?
3. How many subjects were entered? Was the size decided prior to the onset of the study?
4. How were the experimental and control groups selected? Were they selected in a way to ensure equal distribution of known risk factors?
5. Were the treatment regimens described adequately?
   a. If appropriate, was there a nontreated group?
   b. If the control is "standard therapy," was the treatment reasonable?
6. Was this a blinded study?
   a. Did the patients know which treatment they received?
   b. Did the physicians know which treatment patients received?
   c. Did the persons measuring outcome know if patients were in the control or experimental group?
7. What were the results?
   a. Were the treatment groups similar with regard to known prognostic factors?
   b. Were side effects recorded and reported?
   c. Who was included in the final results?
   d. Who was lost to follow-up? Did they differ from those who completed the study?
   e. During analysis, were patients kept in their originally assigned groups?
   f. Were enough of the data presented so that the conclusions can be justified?
   g. Were known risk factors accounted for in the analysis?
   h. Were confidence intervals reported?
   i. If the results were negative, was statistical power addressed?
8. Were the results biologically plausible and consistent with previous literature? If not, was this addressed?

**Table 7–6.** Summary of enrollment criteria for streptokinase-tPA trial.

| Patient Characteristic | Enrolled Subjects |
|---|---|
| Age | < 70 years old |
| Duration of symptoms | < 3 hours |
| Diagnosis | Specific electrocardiographic findings of myocardial infarction |
| Past medical conditions | No history of stroke, bleeding, hypertension, genitourinary bleeding, peptic ulcer confirmed within preceding 6 months; no surgery or trauma within the past 2 weeks; no left bundle branch block or severe noncardiac disease |
| Medications | No current use of anticoagulants |

**Table 7–7.** Possible reasons for noncompliance in a randomized clinical trial.

1. Misunderstanding of instructions.
2. Inconvenience of participation.
3. Side effects of treatment.
4. Cost of participation.
5. Forgetfulness.
6. Disappointment with results.
7. Preference for another treatment.

pliance in a clinical trial (Table 7–8). The investigator may be able to select subjects who can be expected to be compliant. Motivation to participate is likely to be enhanced if the patients perceive themselves to be at high risk of an adverse health consequence. In the streptokinase-tPA trial, for example, all enrolled subjects had just experienced their first myocardial infarction and were no doubt concerned about the possibility of dying. Participants are apt to be motivated to comply also if the treatments offered might reduce the need for painful or debilitating therapy. In the streptokinase-tPA trial, for instance, patients may have hoped that clot lysis would prevent the need for a surgical procedure to bypass the clot.

In nonurgent situations, the investigator may be able to assess probable compliance before randomization is performed. For example, eligible participants may be asked to take either an active or an inert medication in order to monitor compliance. This pretest interval is referred to as a "run-in" test period. Individuals who show a likelihood of compliance then are randomized to the treatments of interest, and those who do not are excluded from the trial. Other strategies to increase compliance include providing incentives for participation or maintaining frequent contact with subjects. Compliance also is likely to be enhanced by keeping the duration of the intervention as brief as possible.

Regardless of how carefully a clinical trial is designed, it is likely that some subjects will not adhere to the treatment regimen. The extent to which participants actually comply can be assessed by a variety of approaches. Personal reports by subjects and family members provide a simple but questionably reliable

**Table 7–8.** Strategies to enhance compliance with treatment assignment in randomized clinical trials.

1. Select motivated persons.
2. Pretest ability and willingness of participants to comply.
3. Provide simple and lucid instructions to subjects.
4. Offer incentives to comply (eg, no charge for therapeutic intervention and associated examinations).
5. Provide positive reinforcements to subjects for adherence to treatment regimen.
6. Maintain frequent contact with participants and remind them about importance of adherence to the regimen.
7. Measure adherence through pill counts or sampling of biologic specimens.
8. Limit duration of intervention.

basis for determining compliance. In drug studies, a traditional approach to assessing compliance is to count the number of unused pills at regular intervals. However, because pills can disappear for reasons other than ingestion by the subject, pill counts provide suggestive but not definitive evidence of compliance. The most conclusive evidence of compliance with a drug regimen is likely to be obtained by measurement of the drug (or a metabolite) in the subject's blood or urine. Even this type of biologic assay has limited utility, however—most obvious constraints being cost, inconvenience to subjects, and the difficulty of collecting specimens from some individuals. Moreover, long-term compliance typically cannot be assessed by measurements of these specimens, since the presence of most drugs is detectable for no more than a few days.

Despite the difficulties inherent in assessing compliance, it is important to estimate the extent to which subjects adhere to the assigned regimens. The ability of a study to identify a true effect of treatment (statistical power) may be diminished if a substantial proportion of the participants do not comply with the assigned treatment. That is, the observed difference in outcomes between the study groups may be reduced because of noncompliance. Accordingly, it may be necessary to include a larger initial sample size to compensate for the loss of discriminatory power. As will be emphasized later in this chapter, it is important to include all randomized patients in the main analysis of a clinical trial. Therefore, every effort should be made to determine the outcomes of both compliant and noncompliant subjects.

## Analysis of Results

Loss of some patients to follow-up is likely to occur in any clinical trial. The more patients lost and the less that is known about them, the less confidence one would place in the results of the trial. In the analysis of results from a clinical trial, *patients should be left in the treatment group originally assigned by the study (intention to treat) even if they received one of the other treatments after the original treatment regimen failed.* In the streptokinase-tPA study, for example, one of the patients received streptokinase and then 9 days later received tPA. The patient subsequently died—but remained in the streptokinase group for purposes of analysis. This may seem counterintuitive, since the patient actually received both treatments. The purpose of this trial, however, was to help clinicians determine the best treatment at the time of initial presentation with myocardial infarction. Subsequent treatment decisions may include the alternative treatment, but those subsequent decisions have no bearing on the original clinical question posed by the trial and thus are not pertinent to group assignment. Design of the streptokinase-tPA trial with consideration of intention to treat is illustrated schematically in Figure 7–5.

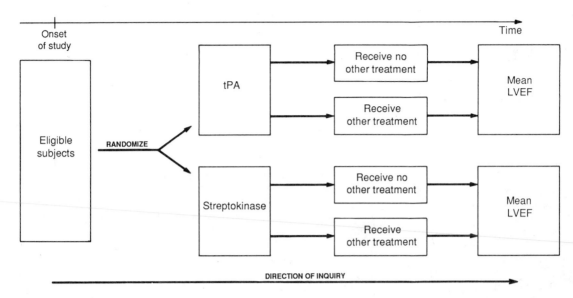

**Figure 7–5.** Schematic diagram of the design of a randomized controlled clinical trial comparing streptokinase with tPA for the treatment of an initial myocardial infarction, with analysis by intention to treat. LVEF = left ventricular ejection fraction.

All participants who are randomized should be included in the analysis of a clinical trial. Selective removal of subjects from the comparison of outcomes, even if it seems justified for pragmatic reasons, may lead to erroneous conclusions. Consider, for example, the question of whether to include noncompliers in the analysis. Since these individuals did not receive the assigned treatments as intended, it may seem illogical to leave them in the analysis. It has been shown, however, that noncompliers tend to have worse outcomes than compliers regardless of their treatment assignment. If the treatment assignment affects the level of compliance, then failure to account for compliance in the analysis can produce a misleading result.

Removal of noncompliers from the analysis may also limit the ability to generalize study findings to clinical practice. In recommending treatment to a particular patient, the physician must consider the possibility that the treatment will not be completed as intended. The essential question of a clinical trial is whether or not a treatment should be offered at a particular point in time. The relevant information on treatment benefit, therefore, is the outcome among all patients who were offered the treatment rather than just those who completed it.

A well-reported clinical trial should contain enough of the primary data to enable the reader (1) to compare the main outcome measure between the treatment groups and (2) to perform basic statistical tests to determine whether chance variation can be reasonably excluded as a cause of observed differences between the groups under comparison. For the clinical trial, it is useful to review three very common

types of comparisons: the comparison of two risks, the comparison of time to an event (survival analysis), and the comparison of two means.

Many outcomes from a clinical trial are yes/no outcomes, (eg, death or no death, cure or no cure, recurrence or no recurrence) and therefore can be displayed in simple tabular format. Early mortality results for patients in the streptokinase-tPA trial are presented in Table 7–9.

The risk of early death in the streptokinase group is the number of deaths within 30 days divided by the total number of streptokinase-treated patients, or 10/135. Similarly, the risk of early death in the tPA group is expressed as 5/135. There are several ways to compare these two risks. Commonly, the two are compared in a ratio, the so-called **risk ratio (*RR*),** or **relative risk** (ie, the risk of early death in one group divided by the risk in the other group). If the *RR* = 1.0, then the risk of the outcome of interest in the two treatment groups is exactly equal. The further the

**Table 7–9.** Results of streptokinase-tPA trial concerning the risk of early death from myocardial infarction.[1]

| Early Death | Treatment | | Total |
|---|---|---|---|
| | **Streptokinase** | **tPA** | |
| Yes | 10 | 5 | 15 |
| No | 125 | 130 | 255 |
| Total | 135 | 135 | 270 |

[1] Adapted and reproduced, with permission, from White HD et al: Effect of intravenous streptokinase as compared with that of tissue plasminogen activator on left ventricular function after myocardial infarction. N Engl J Med 1989;320:817.

ratio is from 1.0, the greater the difference in risk between the two groups. For this trial, the risk of early demise in the streptokinase group compared with the tPA group would be calculated as follows:

$$\text{Risk ratio } (RR) = \frac{10}{135} \bigg/ \frac{5}{135} = 2.0$$

That is, the risk of early death in the streptokinase group is twice that of the tPA group. The value of 2 is referred to as the **point estimate** because it is the single value along the $RR$ scale most consistent with the observed data.

A useful method for gauging the precision of the risk ratio is to calculate the 95% confidence intervals for the $RR$. If the clinical trial was repeated many times, the values that fall between the upper and lower bounds of the 95% confidence interval would include the true $RR$ value 95% of the time. If the 95% confidence interval includes 1.0, then the data are consistent with the null hypothesis and the difference between the groups is not statistically significant at an alpha level of 0.05. If the 95% confidence interval does not include 1.0, then the difference is statistically different at an alpha level of 0.05. The 95% confidence interval (CI) for the streptokinase-to-tPA early risk of death $RR$ calculated above is 0.7 to 5.7. Since the interval includes 1.0, this increased risk is not considered statistically significant at an alpha level of 0.05. This means that the data observed in this trial cannot exclude $RR$ values that range all the way from implying a mild benefit for streptokinase to values that indicate a strong benefit for tPA. The 95% confidence interval for the streptokinase-to-tPA early death $RR$ is illustrated schematically in Figure 7–6. Note that the point estimate of the $RR$ does not lie at the midpoint of the 95% confidence interval. The asymmetry of the confidence interval occurs because the distribution of possible values of the $RR$ is skewed toward the right (ie, all of the values corresponding to a benefit for streptokinase are compressed into the range of zero to 1, whereas the values corresponding

to a benefit for tPA are spread from 1 to positive infinity).

The risk ratio is a simple, easily understood method of evaluating results of clinical trials. For time-to-event data, however, survival analysis has several advantages over the $RR$. The survival curve, as described in Chapter 2, is a graphic presentation of time to an outcome of interest. Since the survival curve graphically depicts events occurring over time, it provides information on the rapidity with which events occur. Furthermore, the survival curve can make use of data from patients who are followed for varying lengths of time. For instance, a trial of drug chemotherapy for cancer patients may be interested in 5-year survival. A patient who is followed for only 3 years provides useful information on survival for that period of time but would provide no information pertinent to a comparison of survival beyond 3 years. Survival analysis also allows one to estimate median survival duration as well as the percentage of survivors at any time along the curve.

An illustration of survival curves for experimental and control groups in a hypothetical randomized clinical trial is shown in Figure 7–7. Time since first treatment is depicted along the horizontal axis, and the percentage of patients remaining alive is displayed on the vertical axis. At the time of initial treatment (years = 0), 100% of the patients in each group are alive. As time from treatment progresses, the percentage of patients who remain alive decreases in both groups, though more rapidly in the control group. At the end of 10 years of follow-up, 45% of the patients treated with the experimental approach remain alive compared with only 20% of the control subjects.

The survival curves could be used to estimate the relative risk of death at any point in time. For example, the experimental-to-control group $RR$ of death at 10 years is as follows:

$$RR = \frac{(100 - 45)}{(100 - 20)} = \frac{55}{80} = 0.69 = 69\%$$

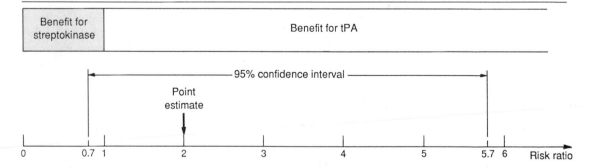

**Figure 7–6.** The point estimate and corresponding approximate 95% confidence interval for the streptokinase-to-tPA early death risk ratio.

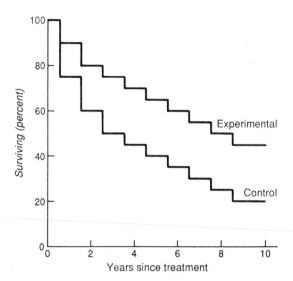

**Figure 7–7.** Survival curves for experimental and control groups in a hypothetical randomized clinical trial.

This *RR* indicates that experimental subjects have about one-third less risk than controls of dying within 10 years. Alternatively, the median survival times for the two groups can be estimated and contrasted. As shown in Figure 7–8, the median survival time is the point at which half of an initial study group remains alive. This time is estimated by drawing a horizontal line at the 50% survival level to each of the survival curves and then drawing vertical lines down to the time axis. In this example, the estimated median survival times are 8 years for the experimental group

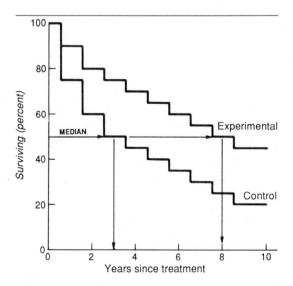

**Figure 7–8.** Approach to estimating median survival times for the experimental and control groups in a hypothetical randomized clinical trial.

and 3 years for the control group. That is, the patients treated with the experimental approach are dying at a slower rate than are the control subjects.

Several tests of significance can be used to compare survival curves (see Dawson-Saunders and Trapp, 1990). It should be noted that although this type of analysis is called survival analysis, it is not limited to the analysis of deaths. Any event that occurs over time—time to disease recurrence, time to return to work, etc—can be compared in this fashion.

Another comparison frequently used in clinical trials is the comparison of means. For example, in the streptokinase-tPA trial, LVEF was chosen as the primary end point. The LVEF is expressed as the percentage of blood ejected from the left ventricle during ventricular contraction and therefore can assume any value between 0 and 100. One could choose to distribute patients into several discrete categories of LVEF (eg, 0–20%, 21–40%, 41–60% . . .), but that would involve a loss of useful information about the actual observed ejection fractions. Instead, the mean or average LVEF can be compared. The null and alternative hypotheses for this comparison would be stated as follows:

$$H_0 : \mu_1 = \mu_2$$

$$H_A : \mu_1 \neq \mu_2$$

A test of the equality of two means can be accomplished by performing a *t* test as follows:

$$t = \frac{\bar{x}_1 - \bar{x}_2}{\left(s_p \sqrt{\dfrac{1}{n_1} + \dfrac{1}{n_2}}\right)}$$

where $\bar{x}_1$ and $\bar{x}_2$ are the observed mean LVEFs of the streptokinase and tPA groups, respectively; $s_p$ is an estimate of the pooled variance of the two means; and $n_1$ and $n_2$ are the sample sizes for each group. To illustrate the use of a *t* test, the LVEFs in patients from the streptokinase-tPA trial who had an anterior myocardial infarction can be compared as follows:

$$t = \frac{(55 - 54)}{15 \sqrt{\dfrac{1}{38} + \dfrac{1}{46}}} = 0.304$$

A *t*-statistic of 0.304 for this sample size corresponds to a *P*-value of 0.762. Since the *P*-value is greater than 0.05, the null hypothesis is not rejected, and one therefore concludes that there is not a statistically significant difference in the means.

Alternatively, the difference between the two means could be calculated by subtraction and a 95% confidence interval constructed around the difference. For the LVEFs mentioned above, the difference between the two groups would be 55 − 54 = 1. The 95% confidence interval for the difference could be calculated (see Dawson-Saunders and Trapp, 1990) and is $-5.51$ to $7.51$. Since the 95% confidence interval contains the null value of 0, the means are not considered to be statistically different at an alpha level of 0.05.

If a study concludes that no difference exists between treatment regimens, then the amount of difference the authors thought was important should be specified as well as the likelihood that the study did not find a difference due to chance alone. The likelihood that a negative result is due to chance is the beta error; 1 minus the beta error $(1 - \beta)$ is the statistical power (see Sample Size Determination).

The reader should interpret the results of a single trial in the context of other clinical trials and other information. If a single trial calls into question previous clinical research or contradicts what is theoretically expected, then additional trials or basic research may be required to help understand the results of the clinical trial.

## SUMMARY

The randomized controlled clinical trial is the most widely accepted approach for comparing the benefits of alternative treatments. The advantages and disadvantages of this research method, as compared with alternative study designs, are set forth in Table 7–10. The principal strength of this approach derives from assigning treatments to patients by randomization, thereby tending to balance the study groups with respect to both known and unknown prognostic factors.

Before enrolling patients in a clinical trial, the investigator can determine the baseline and follow-up information that will be required on all subjects. Procedures then can be put in place to enable the researchers to collect data in a fairly complete and ac-

curate manner. The investigator can also allocate subjects to desired dose levels rather than relying upon physician or patient preferences. When blinding of the evaluators or patients is feasible, the assessment of clinical outcomes is less likely to be influenced by knowing which treatment was used.

Randomized controlled clinical trials are subject to certain constraints, however. Restrictive criteria for inclusion of subjects may produce a very homogeneous study population but at the same time may restrict one's ability to extrapolate results to patients with other characteristics. Clinical trials—particularly those involving chronic processes—may require years of follow-up to determine the outcome of treatment. A prolonged observation period leads to higher costs, increases the likelihood that patients will be lost to follow-up, and delays the time at which a treatment recommendation can be made. The use of intermediate end points, such as LVEF in the streptokinase-tPA trial, can help to limit the length of required follow-up. Nevertheless, a definitive conclusion about treatment benefit often requires years of observation.

Large sample sizes typically are required in clinical trials when the magnitude of difference in responses between study groups is small. Furthermore, large numbers of subjects are likely to be required to demonstrate differences between study groups when there is wide variability in responses to treatment. Increasing the size of the study population not only raises the cost of a trial but may also lead to pragmatic difficulties in locating a sufficiently large pool of eligible patients.

Ethical concerns may arise in a clinical trial if one or more of the treatment options has serious potential side effects. Ethical dilemmas can also arise when early data suggest—but do not establish—therapeutic advantage for one of the treatments. In this situation, a decision must be made about whether the trial should be continued until a definitive conclusion is reached or should be terminated earlier so that all patients have the opportunity to receive the apparently superior treatment. In order to minimize the possible influence of real or perceived conflicts of interest, it is desirable to have an external advisory group review these ethical questions.

An investigator cannot control the behavior of subjects enrolled in a clinical trial. Even after initial informed consent to participate in a clinical trial has been given, a subject has the right to withdraw at any time. Some subjects may elect to remain in the trial but not comply with the assigned regimen. Noncompliance can reduce the statistical power of a clinical trial and thereby lead to a false-negative conclusion. Accordingly, every effort must be made to achieve maximal compliance with assigned treatment without infringing the patient's right to refuse therapy.

**Table 7–10.** Advantages and disadvantages of randomized controlled clinical trials.

**Advantages**
Randomization tends to balance prognostic factors across study groups.
Detailed information can be collected on baseline and subsequent characteristics of participants.
Dose levels can be predetermined by the investigator.
Blinding of participants can reduce distortion in assessment of outcomes.
Assumptions of statistical tests tend to be met.
**Disadvantages**
Subject exclusions may limit ability to generalize findings to other patients.
A long period of time often is required to reach a conclusion.
A large number of participants may be required.
Financial costs are typically high.
Ethical concerns may arise.
Subjects may not comply with treatment assignments.

Ultimately, treatment decisions should be based on the best evidence available concerning therapeutic benefit. The standard approach to gathering this evidence is the randomized controlled clinical trial. Although this type of investigation is labor-intensive, time-consuming, and expensive, it can provide the most convincing evidence of the superiority of one treatment over another. Through the use of randomized clinical trials such as the streptokinase-tPA study, the delivery of patient care can be based upon rigorous scientific information.

## STUDY QUESTIONS

**Directions:** For each question, select the single best answer.

1. A randomized clinical trial was designed to compare two different treatment approaches for asthmatic attacks. The purpose of randomization in this study was to:
   A. Obtain treatment groups of similar size
   B. Select a representative sample of patients for study
   C. Increase patient compliance with treatment
   D. Decrease the likelihood that observed differences in clinical outcome are due to chance
   E. Obtain treatment groups with comparable baseline prognoses

2. In a double-blinded clinical trial concerning the treatment of osteoarthritis, half of the patients received a nonsteroidal anti-inflammatory agent and the other half received a pharmacologically inert substance. Two-thirds of the patients in the former group and one-third of the patients in the latter group reported relief of symptoms. The patients' perceptions of improvement on treatment with an inert substance is best described as:
   A. Intention to treat
   B. Noncompliance
   C. Placebo effect
   D. Type II error
   E. False-positive result

3. In a randomized clinical trial comparing the effectiveness of a new vaccine to that of a standard vaccine for measles, the evaluating clinicians knew which vaccine each patient received but the patients themselves were unaware of the treatment assignment. This design is best described as:
   A. Unblinded
   B. Single-blinded
   C. Double-blinded
   D. Triple-blinded
   E. None of the above

4. The purpose of informed consent in a clinical trial for treatment of hypertension is to:

   A. Increase the patients' knowledge of possible risks and benefits of treatment options
   B. Increase the level of patient participation
   C. Decrease the likelihood of malpractice suits
   D. Decrease the likelihood of a placebo effect
   E. Decrease the likelihood of patient blinding to treatment assignment

5. Which of the following actions is most likely to result in an increase in the statistical power of a clinical trial comparing different weight loss programs?
   A. Blinding of the clinicians who evaluate weight loss
   B. The use of a comparison group that receives only a pharmacologically inert substance
   C. Measurement of patient satisfaction with treatment rather than actual reduction in weight
   D. Increasing the number of patients studied
   E. Restricting the study population to patients with mild obesity

6. A small clinical trial is designed to compare the effectiveness of a new versus a standard chemotherapeutic regimen for the treatment of lymphoma. No difference in 5-year survival percentages is observed despite the fact that in truth, the new treatment is superior. The failure to detect a benefit for the new treatment is best described as:
   A. Observer bias
   B. Placebo effect
   C. Type I error
   D. Type II error
   E. Blinding

7. In a clinical trial comparing medical and surgical treatment of duodenal ulcers, 20% of the patients randomized to medical treatment ultimately underwent a surgical procedure and 10% of the patients initially assigned to surgery later required additional medical management. Analysis of this study according to initial treatment allocation, ignoring subsequent change in therapy, is best described as:
   A. Blinding
   B. Intention to treat
   C. Type I error
   D. Observer bias
   E. Placebo effect

8. In a hospital-based clinical trial of the management of paranoid schizophrenia, relief of symptoms in patients treated with a new drug is compared with symptom relief among patients previously treated with a standard drug. Which of the following is LEAST likely to be a cause of an unfair comparison of the relative benefits of the new and standard drugs?
   A. Changes over time in the criteria used to diagnose paranoid schizophrenia

**B.** Changes over time in the methods used to assess symptom relief

**C.** Changes over time in the nature of patients referred to the hospital

**D.** Inability to blind clinical evaluators to treatment status of patients treated with the new drug

**E.** Lack of use of a separate untreated control group

9. A clinical trial was conducted to evaluate the benefits of an intensive exercise program in reducing subsequent mortality among persons who survive at least 30 days after an initial myocardial infarction. Patients were randomized to receive either usual care (controls) or the exercise program. Among 100 controls, 30 died within the 3-year follow-up period, compared with 50 deaths among the 100 patients on the exercise program. The relative risk of death for the exercise group compared to controls was:

   **A.** 0.20
   **B.** 0.30
   **C.** 0.50
   **D.** 0.60
   **E.** 1.67

10. A randomized clinical trial was undertaken to evaluate the effect of supplemental estrogen in

**Table 7–11.** Baseline characteristics in a randomized clinical trial of the prevention of osteoporosis.

| Characteristic | Level | Experimental | Control |
|---|---|---|---|
| Age (years) | Mean value | 67 | 65 |
| Race | % black | 28 | 24 |
| Body weight | % over ideal | 64 | 42 |
| Calcium supplements | % users | 54 | 60 |
| Exercise | % daily | 46 | 38 |

preventing osteoporosis among postmenopausal women. The experimental group of 50 women received a daily pill of low-dose estrogen, and the control group of 50 women received a placebo. The baseline characteristics of the two groups are shown in Table 7–11. Assuming that each of these characteristics is comparably related to the risk of developing osteoporosis, the factor most likely to contribute to an unfair comparison of experimental and control groups was:

   **A.** Age
   **B.** Race
   **C.** Body weight
   **D.** Calcium supplement use
   **E.** Regular exercise

## FURTHER READING

Buyse MC: Potential and pitfalls of randomized clinical trials in cancer research. Cancer Surv 1989;8:91.

Ratain JS, Hochberg MC: Clinical trials: A guide to understanding methodology and interpreting results. Arth Rheum 1990;33:131.

## REFERENCES

Bull JP: The historical development of clinical therapeutic trials. J Chron Dis 1959;10:218.

Bulpitt CJ: *Randomised Controlled Clinical Trials.* Martinus Nijhoff, 1983.

Dawson-Saunders B, Trapp RG: *Basic and Clinical Biostatistics.* Appleton & Lange, 1990.

Gehlbach SH: *Interpreting the Medical Literature.* 2nd Ed. MacMillan, 1988.

Haygarth J: *Of the Imagination as a Cause and as a Cure of Disorders of the Body.* R. Crutwell, 1801.

Spilker B: *Guide to Clinical Interpretation of Data.* Raven Press, 1986.

White HD et al: Effect of intravenous streptokinase as compared with that of tissue plasminogen activator on left ventricular function after first myocardial infarction. N Engl J Med 1989;320:817.

# Cohort Studies

**8**

## PATIENT PROFILE

*A pediatrician was called to the hospital to attend the delivery of a newborn. The mother was a 28-year-old primigravida and had elevated blood pressure during an otherwise uncomplicated pregnancy. The labor was induced because the pregnancy had continued 2 weeks past the expected date of delivery. There was evidence of fetal distress during labor. When the membranes were ruptured, the obstetrician noted thick greenish fluid containing meconium. At the time of delivery, the male newborn was limp, cyanotic, with no spontaneous respiratory effort, and a heart rate of only 50 beats/min. When an attempt was made to suction meconium from the baby's mouth and nose, there was no grimace, cough, or sneeze.*

*Vigorous efforts at resuscitation were initiated, including bag-and-mask ventilation with 100% oxygen and chest compressions, but the Apgar score at 1 minute of life was 1. The Apgar score (Table 8–1) is an index of neonatal asphyxia and can range from 0 (very asphyxiated) to 10 (no asphyxia). Despite continuing resuscitation, the 5-minute Apgar score had only improved to 2, with the heart rate now at 110 beats/min. The 10-minute Apgar score was 3, and the newborn was transferred to the Newborn Intensive Care Unit. The 3100-g neonate continued to improve with aggressive medical management, without evidence of acute neurologic complications. He was discharged from the hospital on the 12th day of life.*

## CLINICAL BACKGROUND

Perinatal asphyxia can be defined as fetal hypoxia during labor and delivery. Hypoxia in the perinatal period is believed to be a major cause of perinatal deaths as well as of impaired development and neurologic function among survivors. The causes of perinatal asphyxia are not completely understood, but a number of factors, including preeclampsia or eclampsia, maternal hypotension, placental insufficiency, and prematurity, have been associated with hypoxia during labor and delivery. The passage of meconium and the presence of this material in the amniotic fluid indicate possible fetal distress.

The pathogenesis of perinatal asphyxia is presented in Figure 8–1. The development of severe metabolic acidosis in the fetus indicates a lack of oxygen. This is because tissues must resort to anaerobic glycolysis for energy production. The degree of hypoxia a fetus can tolerate before cellular injury occurs is variable and depends on a variety of factors, including previous asphyxia during the pregnancy, metabolic needs versus metabolic reserves, and blood flow to vital organs.

Experimental studies have been performed on newborn primates in which varying degrees of asphyxia were induced. These studies have shown that to produce brain injury, the fetus must be exposed to marked asphyxia for at least 25 minutes. These studies also indicate that this degree of asphyxia will probably lead to fetal death, rather than survival with neurologic impairment. In general, research has shown the immature nervous system to be more resistant to hypoxic injury than the mature brain.

## STUDY DESIGN

The parents of the newborn presented in the Patient Profile are understandably distraught by the unanticipated complications in their baby's first hours of life. Now they have questions about what the future will bring. Will their son develop normal mental capacity? Will he have physical disabilities? Questions like these from concerned parents can often be answered from the pediatrician's own clinical experience. However, it may be that the clinician has seen only a few such patients and must therefore consult the medical literature.

In undertaking such a search, the pediatrician will find a variety of case reports of infants who have had severe perinatal asphyxia and have developed a variety of acute and chronic medical problems. Some of these reports describe dismal outcomes, including death. However, there are reports also of cases of severe asphyxia during delivery followed in later childhood by normal neurologic development and excellent school performance. The pediatrician may then be uncertain about what to tell the parents. Clearly, a broad spectrum of outcomes is possible.

**Table 8–1.** Apgar score for evaluation of neonatal asphyxia.[1,2]

| Sign | Score | | |
|---|---|---|---|
| | **0** | **1** | **2** |
| Heart rate (beats/min) | Absent | <100 | <100 |
| Respiration | Absent | Slow, irregular | Regular, crying |
| Muscle tone | Limp | Slow flexion | Active motor |
| Color | Blue, pale | Body pink, extremities blue | Completely pink |
| Reflex response to catheter in nostril | None | Grimace | Cough, sneeze |

[1]The values for each of the five categories are added to yield a result from 0 to 10.
[2]Adapted with permission, from Apgar V, James LS: Am J Dis Child 1962;104:419 (Copyright 1962, American Medical Association).

What the pediatrician in our example needs to find is a study that offers reliable evidence of the likelihood of each of the various possible outcomes.

The most definitive conclusions could be drawn from a **clinical trial.** This would be a study in which newborns are randomly assigned to different levels of perinatal asphyxia and then followed with measurements of outcome, such as achievement of developmental milestones and school performance. This type of study has actually been performed on laboratory animals, but such a study on human infants would be unethical. An investigator could not intentionally expose humans to potentially harmful conditions simply to learn about the effects on outcome.

Since intentional exposure of human newborns to asphyxia cannot be justified on ethical grounds, the investigator might resort to observing the outcomes of newborns who develop asphyxia under natural circumstances. This type of study is characterized as **observational** because the investigator does not determine the assignment of exposure but rather passively observes events as they unfold. The observational study design that is most similar to the clinical trial is a **cohort study.** In this type of study, as illustrated in Figure 8–2, the investigators identify a population (**cohort**) and determine their initial characteristics (exposure status). A cohort of infants for the purpose of an asphyxia study might consist of infants both with and without perinatal asphyxia. The researchers then follow the cohort over time and determine the outcome in the exposed and unexposed groups. It is important to remember that in a cohort study, information about the risk factor (exposure) is determined prior to the observation of disease status.

A large cohort study was conducted in the United States on the utility of Apgar scores as predictors of chronic neurologic disability. In this study, 49,000 infants were investigated who had Apgar scores recorded at 1 and 5 minutes of age. For those infants who did not achieve a score of 8 or higher at 5 minutes, Apgar scores were also recorded at 10, 15, and 20 minutes. All of the children were then followed to the age of 7 years. The occurrence of seizures was determined through clinical observations in the newborn nursery, and interval histories were recorded at 4, 8, 12, and 18 months of age and yearly thereafter. The presence of cerebral palsy was determined by physical examination at age 7 years. A psychologic and developmental assessment was also performed at age 7. The design of this study is depicted in Figure 8–3.

This study demonstrated that low Apgar scores were a risk factor for the development of cerebral palsy. However, 55% of the children with cerebral palsy at age 7 had Apgar scores of 7 or higher at 1 minute, and 73% scored 7 or higher at 5 minutes. Of the 99 children who survived and had Apgar scores of 0–3 at 10, 15, or 20 minutes, 12 were found to have

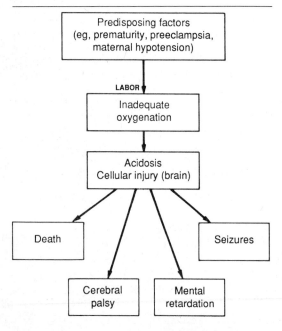

**Figure 8–1.** Schematic representation of the pathogenesis of perinatal asphyxia.

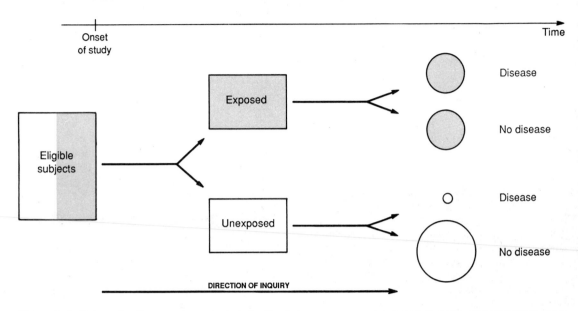

**Figure 8–2.** Schematic diagram of a cohort study. Shaded areas represent exposed persons, and unshaded areas represent unexposed persons.

cerebral palsy. Eleven of those 12 were also mentally retarded. Ten of these infants had seizures in the first 24 hours of life. Of the children who survived and had Apgar scores of 0–3 at 10 minutes or later, 80% were free of any major handicap at early school age.

This study of a large population of children provides the pediatrician in the Patient Profile with the kind of information needed for discussing the baby's prognosis with the parents. It represents an experience that no single practitioner could compile even in a lifetime of practice. The pediatrician can now counsel the parents that although their baby does have an increased risk of cerebral palsy and developmental delay, such an outcome occurs in only about one out

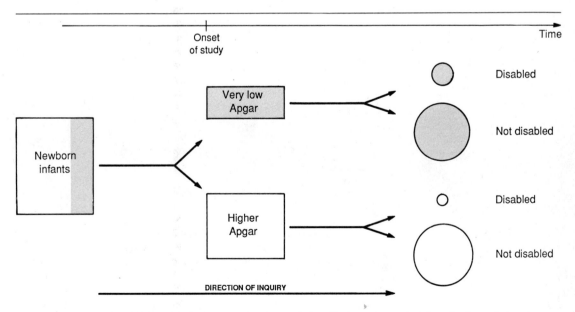

**Figure 8–3.** Schematic diagram of a cohort study of the relationship between perinatal asphyxia and chronic neurologic disability. Shaded areas represent newborns with very low Apgar scores, and unshaded areas represent children with intermediate or high Apgar scores.

of eight asphyxiated neonates. Since the baby did not have a seizure in the first 24 hours of life, the prognosis may be more favorable. It should be reassuring to the parents to learn that 80% of even the most severely asphyxiated newborns were free of major neurologic handicap at early school age.

Perhaps the contributions of cohort studies can be illustrated best by the Framingham Heart Study, one of the most widely recognized and most influential studies of this type. In that investigation, the status of the residents of Framingham, Massachusetts, was determined with respect to potential risk factors for cardiovascular disease. Beginning in 1950, a sample of 6500 individuals aged 30–59 years was chosen from a total population of approximately 10,000 people in that age group. Approximately 5100 subjects with no clinical evidence of atherosclerotic cardiovascular disease agreed to participate in the study. Each subject was examined at the beginning of the study and then reexamined every 2 years. For example, the investigators identified which subjects had elevated blood pressure, which were smokers, and which had elevated serum cholesterol levels. The population then was followed over 35 years to determine which subjects suffered a myocardial infarction, stroke, or other cardiovascular event. This allowed the investigators to determine if an individual with hypertension, for example, was more likely to suffer a stroke than someone who had normal blood pressure.

More than 250 research reports have been produced by the Framingham Heart Study investigators and their collaborators. The Framingham Heart Study is the source of much of our current knowledge about the risk factors for cardiovascular morbidity and mortality. This cohort has also been used to collect information regarding a variety of other diseases.

The Framingham population was chosen for a variety of reasons, including the fact that it was a stable population in which a variety of occupations were represented. The Framingham study is limited, however, because its participants are mainly white, middle-class individuals.

## TIMING OF MEASUREMENTS

A cohort study usually is **prospective,** meaning that the risk factor exposure and subsequent health outcomes are observed after the beginning of the study (Figure 8–2). For example, a prospective cohort study of neonatal asphyxia and subsequent mental retardation could be started in 1993. The degree of birth asphyxia could be determined for births occurring through 1994, and the development of mental retardation could be assessed between 1994 and 1999. An alternative name for such a cohort study is a **longitudinal study.**

Occasionally, a cohort study is **retrospective** (or historical), ie, it utilizes information on prior exposure and disease status. As shown in Figure 8–4, a

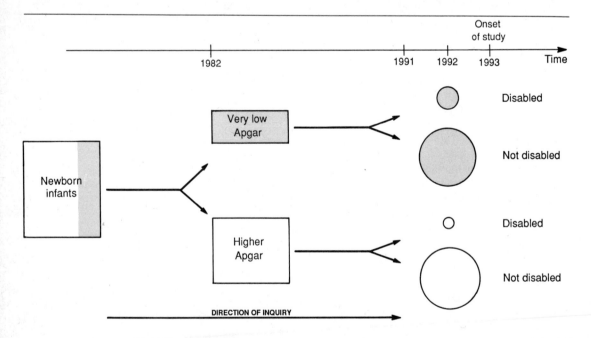

**Figure 8–4.** Schematic diagram of a retrospective cohort study of the relationship between perinatal asphyxia and chronic neurologic disability. Shaded areas represent newborns with very low Apgar scores, and unshaded areas represent children with intermediate or high Apgar scores.

retrospective cohort study of neonatal asphyxia and neurologic disability designed in 1993 might involve a review of the medical records of infants born in a particular hospital in 1982 to determine level of asphyxia, followed by a review of school achievement records over the period 1991–1922 to determine the degree of intellectual functioning. Note that both exposure to risk factors and the subsequent development of the health outcome occur prior to the beginning of the retrospective cohort study.

The advantage of the retrospective cohort design is that all of the events under study have already occurred, and conclusions can therefore be drawn more rapidly. In addition, the cost of a retrospective cohort study might be substantially lower for the same reason. The retrospective approach also may be the only feasible one for studying the effects of exposures that no longer occur, such as discontinued medical treatments. On the other hand, in a retrospective cohort study, one must usually rely upon existing records or subject recall, both of which are usually less complete and accurate than the data collected in a prospective study. Attributes of the prospective and retrospective cohort study designs are compared in Table 8–2.

It should now be clear that a prospective cohort study often takes a long time to complete. Furthermore, in order to have enough subjects developing the outcome of interest to reach a valid conclusion, a cohort study (either prospective or retrospective) usually requires a fairly large number of subjects. For example, in the study of perinatal asphyxia, data concerning 49,000 subjects were accumulated over a 7-year period. This means that such studies can be expensive to complete. In fact, if the disease outcome under study is rare, the sample size required for a cohort study may be so large that it would be impractical to undertake such a study. On the other hand, if the exposure or risk factor is rare, a cohort study may be the most statistically powerful design, because it allows selective inclusion of exposed persons. In the perinatal asphyxia situation, for example, one could include all newborns with Apgar scores of 0–3 but only a sample of the larger pool of newborns with higher scores.

Following subjects over a long period of time can lead to a variety of problems. Subjects may move away or leave the study for other reasons, including death from other causes than the disease under investigation. If the losses to follow-up are substantial, and the lost subjects differ in outcome from those who remain in the study, the validity of the results can be seriously affected. It is also possible for exposure status to change during the course of the study. Obviously, birth asphyxia occurs only once at the beginning of a lifetime. In other circumstances, however, the exposure under study may be subject to variation over time. For example, a cigarette smoker may quit, or, in an occupational cohort study, employees may change jobs and, therefore, their level of exposure to an occupational hazard. Diagnostic methods for the disease under study may also change over time.

The advantages and disadvantages of cohort studies are presented in Table 8–3.

## SELECTION OF SUBJECTS

Selection of subjects for a cohort study is influenced by a variety of factors, including the type of exposure being investigated, the frequency of the exposure in the population, and the accessibility of subjects, as well as the likelihood of their continuing participation. Both the exposed and the unexposed groups must be free of the outcome of interest at the start of the study and equally susceptible to developing the outcome during the course of the study. If some subjects already have the outcome at the onset

**Table 8–2.** Comparison of the attributes of retrospective and prospective cohort studies.

| Attribute | Retrospective Approach | Prospective Approach |
|---|---|---|
| Information | Less complete and accurate | More complete and accurate |
| Discontinued exposures | Useful | Not useful |
| Emerging, new exposures | Not useful | Useful |
| Expense | Less costly | More costly |
| Completion time | Shorter | Longer |

**Table 8–3.** Advantages and disadvantages of cohort studies.

| Advantages | Disadvantages |
|---|---|
| Direct calculation of risk ratio (relative risk) | Time-consuming |
| May yield information on the incidence of disease | Often requires a large sample size |
| Clear temporal relationship between exposure and disease | Expensive |
| Particularly efficient for study of rare exposures | Not efficient for the study of rare diseases |
| Can yield information on multiple exposures | Losses to follow-up may diminish validity |
| Can yield information on multiple outcomes of a particular exposure | Changes over time in diagnostic methods may lead to biased results |
| Minimizes bias | |
| Strongest observational design for establishing cause-and-effect relationship | |

of the study, the temporal relationship between the exposure and the disease will be obscured.

## The Exposed Group

The type of exposure under investigation is critical for selection of the exposed group. Some exposures during pregnancy are common, such as gestational diabetes or hypertension. For these exposures, a general population of pregnancies could be used to construct the cohort. Other exposures, such as in vitro fertilization, are not common among all pregnant women. In order to evaluate whether in vitro fertilization is a risk factor for developmental disability in the offspring through a cohort study design, it may be necessary to sample exposed subjects from an infertility clinic rather than from among pregnant women in the general population.

Feasibility issues are also important when selecting the exposed population. The investigator should identify an accessible population that is motivated to participate in the study and unlikely to discontinue participation. The availability of historical information such as medical records may also be a factor in selecting this group. Examples of groups that have been chosen for feasibility reasons include nurses, members of health maintenance organizations, stable communities, and labor union members.

The degree of exposure may differ depending on the goals of the study. For some exposures, subjects are classified simply into two groups: exposed and unexposed. In vitro fertilization is an example of this type of dichotomization. Other studies involve a range of exposure levels, eg, Apgar scores as an indicator of perinatal asphyxia. The investigator may take a graded exposure variable, such as the Apgar score, and transform it into a categorical exposure by dividing the subjects into those who exceed a certain designated value (eg, Apgar score of 3) and those who are below that value. The value chosen to separate groups is referred to as a **cutoff point** and can be selected in various ways. For example, it might be selected on the basis of the underlying distribution of values, such as the point that separates the 10% of subjects with the lowest Apgar scores from the remainder of the population. Alternatively, one can use a standard cutoff point believed to have pathophysiologic implications regardless of the underlying distribution in the population.

Thus, Apgar scores can be classified into dichotomous categories (0–3 versus > 3), into multiple ordered categories (0–3, 4–6, 7–10), or by gradations (continuous). If the exposure can be categorized into multiple levels or gradations, the investigator can determine whether a relationship exists between the dose of the exposure and the response. In the present context, for example, one can address the question whether the risk of chronic neurologic disability rises as the Apgar score decreases. If such a trend is observed, the argument that perinatal asphyxia is a cause of chronic neurologic disability is strengthened.

## The Unexposed Group

The feasibility issues for the unexposed group are similar to those that apply to the exposed group. The unexposed group must be accessible for entry into the study and for follow-up. When the purpose of the cohort study is to investigate a community, such as in the Framingham Heart Study, the source of the unexposed persons is the community. Since there may be more unexposed persons in the community than are needed for the investigation, a representative sample may be taken. In the Framingham Heart Study, several risk factors were of interest, all of which were relatively prevalent in the community. In this situation, a sample of the entire community was drawn and then subdivided into exposure groups depending upon the risk factor of interest in a particular analysis. In the study of perinatal asphyxia, the unexposed group was defined as the infants with the highest Apgar scores (7–10), indicating the lowest degree of perinatal asphyxia.

For cohort studies that involve the selection of a specific exposed population, selection of an appropriate comparison population may be less clear-cut. For example, if one is studying in vitro fertilization as a risk factor for congenital malformations, the comparison group might be pregnant women who are followed in other obstetric practices. However, if the comparison pregnancies are not followed with a comparable level of clinical scrutiny—or if they differ from the exposed pregnancies in other ways that might be related to congenital malformations—then the study may lead to a false conclusion. The investigator may relate the risk of congenital malformation to in vitro fertilization when in fact it was due to some other difference between the exposed and unexposed groups. This type of problem illustrates why a randomized controlled clinical trial may be less susceptible to error than a cohort study. With randomization, factors known to be related to the development of disease—as well as other factors not yet recognized as related to the disease—tend to be balanced between the groups. This justifies confidence that an observed association is in fact due to the exposure of interest rather than to some other characteristic.

The underlying principle in selecting the unexposed group is that it should yield a fair comparison with the exposed group. Occasionally, the frequency of outcome occurrence in the exposed population is compared with the outcome frequency in the general population. This is particularly useful when members of the general population are very unlikely to be exposed to the study factor. However, the general population may not be comparable with those in the exposed group. For example, follow-up for disease occurrence may be more (or less) complete than for the exposed study group. This may lead to erroneous conclusions. Furthermore, if the exposed and unexposed groups are chosen from different time periods (nonconcurrent study), medical care or other factors may differ between the groups in a way that makes the comparison unfair and the results invalid. Suggestions for the selection of exposed and unexposed subjects are presented in Table 8–4.

## DATA COLLECTION

The investigator must collect information on both the independent variable (exposure) and the dependent variable (response) during the course of a cohort study.

### Exposure

It is essential to define the exposure clearly. Some exposures are acute, one-time episodes, never repeated in a subject's lifetime, eg, asphyxia at birth. Other exposures are long-term, such as cigarette smoking or the use of oral contraceptives. Exposures may also be intermittent, eg, pregnancy-induced hypertension, which may occur during one pregnancy, disappear after delivery, and perhaps reappear during subsequent pregnancies. The types of exposure characteristics that should be considered are presented in Table 8–5.

A subject who originally satisfies the criteria for inclusion in a cohort study should not be excluded from the analysis subsequently because of a change in exposure status during follow-up. This type of exclusion may lead to a biased conclusion. Specifically, it is possible that a change in exposure status may indicate a change in outcome status. For example, in studying the relationship between the use of an antinausea medication during pregnancy and subsequent risk of spontaneous abortion, the use of the medication may be discontinued because of early signs of threatened abortion. Excluding this subject from the analysis, therefore, may result in an underestimate of

**Table 8–5.** Measurements of exposure used in cohort studies. (*Example:* gestational hypertension.)

| Measurements of Exposure | Examples |
| --- | --- |
| Intensity | Mean blood pressure level |
| Duration | Weeks of hypertension |
| Regularity | Number of affected pregnancies |
| Variability | Range of measured blood pressures |

the true link between the medication and the risk of abortion. The potential for changes in exposure status does have important implications for the frequency of follow-up. Frequent reassessment of exposure as well as outcome status may be required if exposure status changes over time.

The source of available information about exposure may constrain the ability of the investigator to define and measure exposure experience. If the information comes from medical records, as is sometimes necessary in a retrospective cohort study, the quality of exposure information may be poor. For example, there are inherent disadvantages in using Apgar scores from medical records. The Apgar scoring system can be subjective and is sometimes recoded by the medical staff as part of the required paperwork some time after delivery. Furthermore, the score may not have been assessed precisely at 1, 5, or 10 minutes. In the previously cited prospective cohort study of neonatal asphyxia, a specially trained independent observer who was not responsible for patient care recorded the score in a standard manner on a standardized study form at exactly 1, 5, and 10 minutes of life.

In general, objective measures of exposure or biologic markers of exposure are preferred over subjective measures. For example, in a study of maternal use of illicit drugs and pregnancy outcome, one approach to exposure assessment would be to question pregnant women about their use of illicit drugs. Self-reports of illicit drug use, however, are likely to underrepresent actual exposure. Repeated measurements of drug metabolites in urine might provide a more accurate and reliable assessment of exposure.

### Clinical Response

Before the start of the study, it is imperative to determine that the subjects do not have the outcome (disease) being investigated. This may be especially difficult if the outcome is a disease that develops slowly, has an insidious onset, and is asymptomatic until its late stages. One approach to this problem is to exclude cases that emerge early in the course of the

**Table 8–4.** Guidelines for selection of exposed and unexposed subjects in cohort studies.

Unexposed persons should be sampled from the same (or comparable) source population as the exposed group.
Both exposed and unexposed groups should be free of the disease of interest and equally susceptible to development of the disease at the beginning of the study.
The baseline characteristics of exposed persons should not differ systematically from those of unexposed persons except for the exposure of interest.
Equivalent information (quantity and quality) should be available on exposure and disease status in the exposed and unexposed groups.
Both groups should be accessible and available for follow-up.
Multiple comparison groups of unexposed subjects chosen in different ways may reinforce the validity of findings.

investigation under the assumption that the onset of disease preceded the beginning of the study.

The degree of surveillance for disease should be similar in the exposed and unexposed groups. The frequency of examination and the duration of follow-up depend on the type of exposure and the outcome under investigation. For some diseases, the time from exposure to development of disease is short. A cohort study of the relationship between exposure to peri-natal asphyxia and death within the first week of life, for example, would have a short follow-up period. Other outcomes, such as chronic neurologic dis-ability, may require years to assess. The study of the relationship of perinatal asphyxia to neurologic devel-opment required follow-up for 7 years because the investigators were interested in performance and cog-nitive ability at early school age.

The information on outcome status may come from a variety of sources. Some cohort studies rely on information from physician and hospital records. This would be particularly pertinent for a cohort study focusing on a population with good access to health care and standardized record-keeping practices, such as a prepaid health plan. Other cohort studies may combine physician records with periodic examina-tions by the investigators. The Framingham Heart Study is an example of this type of study. Another approach to collecting information on disease is to have the subjects themselves report whether or not they develop the outcome. The study may also in-volve reviews of medical records in a subset of sub-jects to confirm the self-reports.

If the outcome under study is death from any cause, the investigator may use information from death certificates. However, death certificates may not be useful if the study is focusing on a specific disease, since cause-of-death information on death certificates may be inaccurate. Obviously, the best information in that circumstance would come from autopsy reports. Since most people who die are not autopsied, however, this may not be feasible.

If diagnostic evaluations are performed by the in-vestigator during the course of the study, there must be an appropriate diagnostic test for the disease (see Chapter 6). This approach has limitations because diagnostic tests are not always available or feasible. In order to ensure a fair comparison between the ex-posed and unexposed groups, the accuracy and re-liability of diagnosis must not differ between these two groups. It can be helpful if those who assess outcomes are unaware of the subjects' exposure sta-tus. The study of perinatal asphyxia relied on stan-dard neurologic examination as well as psychologic tests. The examiners had no access to the medical records and thus were blind to the Apgar scores of the children. This should facilitate an assessment of neu-rologic outcomes that is comparable for exposed and unexposed children.

It is possible for the exposure status to alter the surveillance for disease. An example of this problem could occur in a study of neonatal asphyxia and intel-lectual development. If a physician is more likely to administer psychologic and developmental tests to an infant who had a difficult birth with low Apgar scores, that child is more apt to be diagnosed as hav-ing subtle developmental problems than another child not singled out for close surveillance. This could lead to an overestimate of the relationship between neonatal asphyxia and subsequent developmental dis-ability. This problem can be avoided, as in the cited study, by ensuring that a standard diagnostic protocol is adhered to regardless of exposure status.

## ANALYSIS

Several different approaches can be used to analyze the results of a cohort study, as described in the fol-lowing sections.

### Risk Ratio

The results of a cohort study can be summarized in the format shown in Table 8–6. In this table, the letters A–D represent numbers of subjects in the four possible combinations of exposure and outcome sta-tus (in this instance, death).

A. Exposed persons who later die
B. Unexposed persons who later die
C. Exposed persons who do not die
D. Unexposed persons who do not die

The total number of subjects in this study is the sum of A + B + C + D. The total number of exposed persons is A + C, and the total number of unexposed persons is B + D.

Among exposed persons, the risk ($R$) of death is defined as:

$$R_{(exposed)} = \frac{\text{Exposed persons who die}}{\text{All exposed persons}}$$

$$= \frac{A}{A + C}$$

As indicated in Chapter 2, risk can vary between 0 (no exposed persons die) and 1 (all exposed persons die). As in all statements of risk, some time period for

**Table 8–6.** Summary of risk data from a cohort study.

| Outcome[1] | Exposed | Unexposed | Total |
|---|---|---|---|
| Death | A | B | A + B |
| No death | C | D | C + D |
| Total | A + C | B + D | A + B + C + D |

[1] In some studies, the outcome is development of disease rather than death.

the development of the outcome must be specified. For example, the outcome might be the risk of death in the first year of life. Among unexposed persons, the risk of death is defined as:

$$R_{(unexposed)} = \frac{\text{Unexposed persons who die}}{\text{All unexposed persons}}$$

$$= \frac{B}{B + D}$$

As indicated in Chapters 4 and 7, one approach to contrasting the risk in two groups is to create a ratio measure. The **risk ratio** (*RR*), or relative risk, is:

$$RR = \frac{R_{(exposed)}}{R_{(unexposed)}} = \frac{A/(A + C)}{B/(B + D)}$$

If the exposed and unexposed persons have the same risk of death, then the *RR* is 1 (ie, the null value). That is, exposure is not related to the outcome. If the risk among exposed persons is greater than the corresponding risk among unexposed persons, then the *RR* is greater than 1 (ie, hazardous exposure). In contrast, if the risk among exposed persons is smaller than the corresponding risk among unexposed persons, then the *RR* is less than 1 (ie, beneficial exposure).

The calculation of risk ratio can be illustrated from the study of perinatal asphyxia. The data in Table 8–7 relate to infants who weighed more than 2500 g at birth. Exposure is defined as an Apgar score of 0–3 at 10 minutes of life, and the comparison group of less exposed newborns had Apgar scores of 4–6 at 10 minutes. In the actual study, a third group with Apgar scores of 7–10 was included, but the data are not described here in detail.

The risk among exposed newborns is:

$$R_{(exposed)} = \frac{42}{122} = 0.344 = 34.4\%$$

That is, about one out of three newborns weighing more than 2500 g with very low Apgar scores at 10 minutes died during the first year of life. The risk among "less exposed" newborns is:

**Table 8–7.** Relationship between 10-minute Apgar scores and risk of death in the first year of life among children with birth weights of at least 2500 g.[1]

|  | Apgar Score 0–3 | Apgar Score 4–6 | Total |
|---|---|---|---|
| Death | 42 | 43 | 85 |
| No death | 80 | 302 | 382 |
| Total | 122 | 345 | 467 |

[1] Data used, with permission, from Nelson KB, Ellenberg JH: Apgar scores as predictors of chronic neurologic disability. Pediatrics 1981;68:36.

$$R_{(less\ exposed)} = \frac{43}{345} = 0.125 = 12.5\%$$

In other words, one in eight neonates weighing over 2500 g with intermediate Apgar scores at 10 minutes died during the first year of life.

Without any further calculations, it should be obvious that the neonates with very low 10-minute Apgar scores had a worse prognosis than those with intermediate 10-minute Apgar scores. Quantification of the magnitude of this effect is achieved by calculating the risk ratio:

$$RR = \frac{42}{122} \Big/ \frac{43}{345} = 2.8$$

The *RR* of 2.8 means that newborns at this birth weight with very low 10-minute Apgar scores are almost three times more likely to die in the first year of life as are newborns with intermediate 10-minute Apgar scores. The *RR* is a measure of the strength of association between exposure and outcome. The further the *RR* is away from the null value of 1, the stronger the association. The strength of association is an important criterion in evaluating whether an observed association is likely to represent a cause-and-effect relationship. The *RR* of 2.8 is consistent with a moderate to strong relationship between the exposure (10-minute Apgar score) and outcome (infant death).

As discussed in Chapter 7, a sense of the statistical precision of this estimated risk ratio can be obtained by calculating **confidence intervals** around the point estimate of 2.8. Using the approximation method described in Appendix C, the 95% confidence interval for the data presented in Table 8–7 is (1.9, 4.1). That is, at the 95% level of confidence, the range of *RR* values consistent with the observed data fall between 1.9 and 4.1. Thus, the data indicate a risk of death in infants with very low Apgar scores that ranges between roughly a doubling and a fourfold increase (Figure 8–5). As demonstrated in Chapter 7, the point estimate does not lie in the middle of the *RR* confidence interval. The asymmetry of this interval derives from the skew of the range of values of the risk ratio toward the positive direction (ie, all beneficial effects are compressed into the range 0–1, whereas hazardous effects range from 1 to positive infinity).

Since the null value is excluded from this 95% confidence interval, one can conclude that the findings are **statistically significant.** In other words, these data are not consistent with the null hypothesis of no association between Apgar scores and infant mortality (at the prespecified 95% level of confidence). An association as strong as that observed between Apgar scores and infant mortality, therefore, cannot be explained by chance alone.

As indicated earlier, the argument that the linkage between Apgar score and death in the first year of life is one of cause and effect is strengthened if a dose-

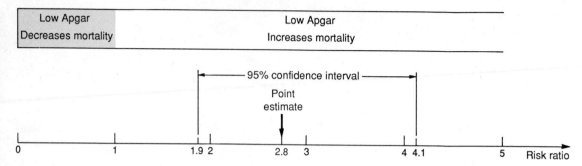

**Figure 8–5.** Point estimate and 95% confidence interval for risk ratio comparing infant mortality in newborns weighing more than 2500 g with 10-minute Apgar scores of 0–3 to that of newborns with 10-minute Apgar scores of 4–6.

response relationship can be demonstrated. A third group of newborns, with Apgar scores of 7–10, was therefore included in the study. Comparison of the risk of death in that group against the previously used reference group with intermediate Apgar scores of 4–6 yields a risk ratio of 0.15, with an approximate 95% confidence interval of (0.11, 0.21). This result means that newborns with a 10-minute Apgar score of 7–10 have only about one-sixth the risk of death in the first year of life as do newborns with Apgar scores of 4–6. This disparity is statistically significant, and the very narrow width of the confidence interval indicates a statistically precise estimate (because it is based upon a large number of observations).

The dose-response relationship between Apgar score and the risk ratio of death in the first year of life for newborns weighing more than 2500 g is shown in Figure 8–6. The reference group against which others were compared in the preceding calculations was the group with Apgar scores of 4–6 (ie, the risk ratio for this group is defined as 1). A clear trend of decreasing risk ratio with increasing Apgar score is seen, and this trend is unlikely to have occurred by chance alone. Thus, there is strong evidence in these data for a dose-response relationship.

## Attributable Risk Percent

The risk of a specified outcome can be compared with measures other than a ratio. For example, one can simply subtract the risk for one group from that of another. This measure is termed the **risk difference,** or excess risk. Some authors use the term "attributable risk" for this measure, but that expression is discouraged here because it may be confused with other expressions. The risk difference (*RD*) is defined as:

$$RD = R_{(exposed)} - R_{(unexposed)}$$

$$= \frac{A}{A + C} - \frac{B}{B + D}$$

Using the previously cited data relating 10-minute Apgar scores (0–3 versus 4–6) to the risk of death in the first year of life, the risk difference is:

$$RD = \frac{42}{122} - \frac{43}{345} = 0.344 - 0.125 = 0.219$$

That is, the risk of death in the first year of life is increased by 0.219 for newborns weighing more than 2500 g who have a 10-minute Apgar score of 0–3 compared with those with a 10-minute Apgar score of 4–6.

Another measure of interest is the **attributable risk percent** (*ARP*), in which the risk difference is expressed as a percentage of the total risk experienced by the exposed group:

$$ARP = \frac{R_{(exposed)} - R_{(unexposed)}}{R_{(exposed)}} \times 100$$

$$= \frac{A/(A + C) - B/(B + D)}{A/(A + C)} \times 100$$

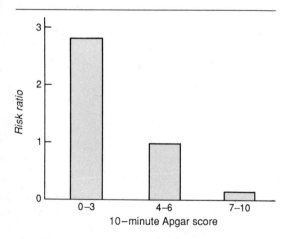

**Figure 8–6.** Dose-response relationship for the association between 10-minute Apgar scores and risk of death in the first year of life among newborns with a birth weight over 2500 g. (Data used, with permission, from Nelson KB, Ellenberg JH: Apgar scores as predictors of chronic neurologic disability. Pediatrics 1981;68:36.)

For the Apgar score-infant mortality data, the attributable risk percent is:

$$ARP = \frac{(0.344 - 0.125)}{0.344} \times 100 = 63.7\%$$

In other words, almost two-thirds of the total risk of infant mortality for newborns weighing more than 2500 g with 10-minute Apgar scores of 0–3 is related to an Apgar score below the 4–6 level. The attributable risk percent typically is used as an indicator of the public health impact of exposure. These data suggest that birth asphyxia is a major contributor to but not the sole cause of infant mortality among severely asphyxiated children.

## Rate Ratio

The analyses presented thus far are based upon comparisons of risk estimates across exposure groups. In a cohort study, the measured outcome may be an incidence (or mortality) rate rather than a risk. The format used to summarize rate data in a cohort study is presented in Table 8–8. The rate ratio is derived as follows:

$$\text{Rate ratio} = \frac{\text{Rate of outcome among exposed persons}}{\text{Rate of outcome among unexposed persons}}$$
$$= \frac{A/PT_{(exposed)}}{B/PT_{(unexposed)}}$$

The magnitude of the rate ratio is interpreted in the same manner as the risk ratio ($< 1$ = protective effect, $1$ = no effect, $> 1$ = harmful effect of exposure). The further away from the null value, the stronger the association between exposure and the rate of the outcome.

The data collected in the study of perinatal asphyxia were not presented in a manner that allows calculation of rate ratios.

In order to illustrate this measure, then, data are drawn from the Chicago Heart Association Detection Project in Industry (Dyer et al, 1992). That investigation involved almost 40,000 men and women at 84 cooperating companies and institutions in the Chicago area. Subjects were enrolled between 1967 and 1973, screened for cardiovascular disease risk factors, and then followed an average of 14–15 years. For white males aged 25–39 at entry, the relationship between baseline serum cholesterol and subsequent rate of coronary heart disease (CHD) is shown in Table 8–9. The rate ratio is:

$$\text{Rate ratio} = \frac{26/36,581}{14/68,239} = 3.5$$

In other words, the CHD mortality rate among white males with borderline high cholesterol levels was about three and one-half times higher than that of white males with lower cholesterol levels. Adjustment for underlying age differences in the study groups reduced the observed rate ratio to 3.1. Comparison of CHD mortality among white males 25–39 with high serum cholesterol levels ($> 6.2$ mmol/L [$> 240$ mg/dL]) to those with normal levels ($\leqslant 5.1$ mmol/L [$\leqslant 197$ mg/dL]) yielded an age-adjusted rate ratio of 5.1. Thus, a dose-response relationship was evident between baseline serum cholesterol level and subsequent CHD mortality.

## SUMMARY

In this chapter, the basic approach to the design and analysis of cohort studies was presented, with illustrations drawn primarily from the literature on birth asphyxia. A cohort study is a type of observational investigation in which subjects are classified on the basis of level of exposure to a risk factor and then followed to determine subsequent disease outcome. **Prospective** cohort studies are conducted by making all observations on exposure and disease status after the onset of the investigation. A **retrospective** cohort study involves observations on exposure and disease status prior to the onset of the study. The retrospective approach offers several pragmatic advantages but may result in less accurate and complete information on exposure and disease status.

Cohort studies are statistically efficient for the study of rare exposures because the exposed individuals can be selectively included in the study. On the

Table 8–8. Summary format of rate data from a cohort study.

| | Exposed Persons | Unexposed Persons | Total |
|---|---|---|---|
| Number of outcomes | $A$ | $B$ | $A + B$ |
| Person-time ($PT$) | $PT_{(exposed)}$ | $PT_{(unexposed)}$ | $PT_{(total)}$ |

Table 8–9. Relationship between baseline serum cholesterol level and subsequent coronary heart disease mortality rate among white males aged 25–39 at entry into the Chicago Heart Association Study.[1]

| | Cholesterol Level | | |
|---|---|---|---|
| | 5.2–6.2 mmol/L[2] | ≤5.1 mmol/L[3] | Total |
| Deaths | 26 | 14 | 40 |
| Person-years | 36,581 | 68,239 | 104,820 |

[1] Data from Dyer AR, Stamler J, Shekelle RB: Serum cholesterol and mortality from coronary heart disease in young, middle-aged, and older men and women from three Chicago epidemiologic studies. Ann Epidemiol 1992;2:51.
[2] 201–240 mg/dL.
[3] ≤ 197 mg/dL.

other hand, cohort studies are inefficient for the investigation of slowly developing or rare diseases. The evaluation of chronic diseases through the cohort approach requires a long follow-up period and increases the chances that subjects will be lost from the study. The evaluation of rare diseases with the cohort study approach requires a large sample size and therefore is expensive and labor-intensive.

There are several basic strategies for the analysis of cohort studies. If data are collected on the risk of developing the outcome during some specified period of time, then the summary measure of effect typically is the **risk ratio,** or the risk of the outcome among exposed subjects divided by the risk of the outcome among unexposed ones. An alternative approach to contrasting risks is the **risk difference,** which is the risk among exposed minus the risk among unexposed. If the risk difference is divided by the risk among exposed, a measure termed the **attributable risk percent** is derived. The attributable risk percent is an indicator of the proportion of risk that may be attributable to the exposure per se. When the data in a cohort study are based upon the rate of disease outcome, the standard measure of effect is the **rate ratio.** The checklist provided in Table 8–10 may serve as a useful guide in evaluating the design and the analysis of published cohort studies.

The prospective cohort study of perinatal asphyxia cited in this chapter indicated that Apgar scores can serve as a useful predictor of subsequent risk of death and neurologic disability. There is an inverse dose-response relationship between Apgar score level and the risk of adverse neurologic outcome. In spite of this increased risk, however, most children with low Apgar scores survive and do not manifest neurologic or developmental disability. Through proper interpretation of the results of this cohort study, the pediatrician in the Patient Profile can inform the baby's parents that although their child faces an increased risk of certain disabilities, there is about an 80% chance that no neurologic handicaps will develop.

## STUDY QUESTIONS

**Directions:** For each question, select the single best answer.

**Questions 1–3:** A retrospective cohort study is conducted of the relationship between perimenopausal exogenous estrogen use and the risk of coronary heart disease. A total of 5000 exposed and 5000 unexposed women are enrolled and followed for 15 years for the development of myocardial infarction. A total of 200 estrogen users developed the outcome compared with 300 myocardial infarctions among the nonusers.

1. The risk of a myocardial infarction among estrogen users is:
   A. 0.02
   B. 0.04

**Table 8–10.** Checklist for the evaluation of published cohort studies.

**Hypothesis**
A. Is the study hypothesis clearly stated?
B. Does it address a question of clinical interest and importance?
**Design**
A. Is the cohort design appropriate for the question to be answered?
B. Is it feasible to perform a cohort study?
**Study population**
A. Will the study yield a fair comparison between the exposed and unexposed subjects?
B. Is the sample size adequate to answer the question of interest?
C. Do the exposed and unexposed subjects come from the same or different populations?
D. Are the exposed and unexposed subjects examined concurrently?
E. Does the investigator present a rationale for the choice of study population?
F. Is the study population similar to the type seen in clinical practice?
**Exposure**
A. Has the exposure been defined?
B. What is the source of exposure information?
C. Has the exposure been measured appropriately?
D. Are there objective measures or markers to substantiate subjective measures?
E. Is the exposure an acute or chronic one?
F. For chronic exposures, is there remeasurement during the course of the study?
G. Is it possible to examine a dose-response relationship?
**Disease**
A. Is the disease clearly defined?
B. What is the source of information about the disease?
C. Is there pathologic or other confirmation of disease?
D. Has the presence of disease been assessed in a similar fashion for the exposed and unexposed groups?
E. Were those who assessed disease status blind to subject exposure status?
**Follow-up**
A. Was the period of follow-up adequate for the development of disease?
B. Were appropriate measures taken to maintain subjects in the study?
C. Is there discussion of losses to follow-up?
**Analysis**
A. Was an appropriate analysis performed?
B. Are the results statistically significant?
C. Are the results clinically meaningful?

   C. 0.06
   D. 0.67
   E. 1.50

2. The risk of a myocardial infarction among non-users of estrogen is:
   A. 0.02
   B. 0.04
   C. 0.06
   D. 0.67
   E. 1.50

3. The risk ratio of a myocardial infarction is:
   A. 0.02
   B. 0.04

C. 0.06
D. 0.67
E. 1.50

**Questions 4–5:** A prospective cohort study is conducted of the relationship between visual impairment and the risk of injuries from falls among the elderly. A total of 400 visually impaired persons aged 70 or older are compared against 400 persons of comparable age without visual impairment. Over a 5-year follow-up period, 80 visually impaired persons have injuries from falls and 20 non-visually impaired persons have injuries from falls.

4. The risk difference is:
   A. 0.05
   B. 0.10
   C. 0.15
   D. 0.20
   E. 0.50

5. The attributable risk percent is:
   A. 15%
   B. 20%
   C. 50%
   D. 67%
   E. 75%

**Questions 6–7:** A prospective cohort study is conducted of the relationship between alcohol consumption and the rate of breast cancer development. A total of 2000 women who consume moderate levels of alcohol are followed for an average of 10 years. The comparison group consists of 2000 nondrinking women who also are followed for 10 years on average. A total of 30 newly diagnosed breast cancers developed among moderate drinkers, and 15 breast cancers were diagnosed among nondrinkers.

6. The incidence rate (per 10,000 woman-years) of breast cancer among moderate drinkers is:
   A. 15
   B. 30

C. 45
D. 60
E. 300

7. The rate ratio of breast cancer is:
   A. 0.3
   B. 0.5
   C. 1.0
   D. 2.0
   E. 3.0

**Questions 8–9:** In a retrospective cohort study of occupational exposure to a particular pesticide, the risk ratio for development of lymphoma is 2.0, with a 95% confidence interval of (0.8, 4.0).

8. The point estimate of the *RR* suggests that the effect of pesticide exposure upon risk of lymphoma is:
   A. To increase risk
   B. Unrelated to risk
   C. To decrease risk
   D. Only related to risk under certain conditions

9. At the 5% level of significance, the association between pesticide exposure and risk of lymphoma is:
   A. Statistically significant
   B. Not statistically significant
   C. Of uncertain statistical significance without a hypothesis test
   D. Not appropriately assessed by statistical significance because randomization was not performed

10. Each of the following is likely to be an advantage of retrospective as opposed to prospective cohort studies EXCEPT
    A. Less expensive
    B. More rapidly completed
    C. Useful for the evaluation of discontinued medical treatments
    D. Allows more accurate assessment of exposure

## FURTHER READING

Feinleib M, Breslow NE, Detels R: Cohort studies. In: *Oxford Textbook of Public Health*, 2nd ed, Vol 2. Holland WW, Detels R, Knox G (editors). Oxford Univ Press, 1991.

## REFERENCES

### Study Design

Feinleib M: The Framingham Study: Sample selection, follow-up, and methods of analysis. In: *National Cancer Institute Monograph*, No. 67. Greenwald P (editor). US Department of Health and Human Services, 1985.

Nelson KB, Ellenberg JH: Apgar scores as predictors of chronic neurologic disability. Pediatrics 1981;68:36.

**Timing of Measurements**

Greenberg RS: Prospective studies. In: *Encyclopedia of Statistical Sciences,* Vol 7. Kotz S, Johnson NL (editors). Wiley, 1986.

Greenberg RS: Retrospective studies (including case-control). In: *Encyclopedia of Statistical Sciences,* Vol 8. Kotz S, Johnson NL (editors). Wiley, 1988.

**Analysis**

Dyer AR, Stamler J, Shekelle RB: Serum cholesterol and mortality from coronary heart disease in young, middle-aged, and older men and women in three Chicago epidemiologic studies. Ann Epidemiol 1992;2:51.

Kleinbaum DG, Kupper LL, Morgenstern H: *Epidemiologic Research*. Lifetime Learning, 1982.

# Case-Control Studies

9

## PATIENT PROFILE

*A 10-year-old girl had been in excellent health until 2 weeks before presentation, when she developed a viral upper respiratory illness with malaise, rhinorrhea, temperature of 38 °C, and cough. After taking aspirin, she felt better and her temperature returned to normal. However, after several days she became sleepy, vomited, and, because of her worsening condition, was taken to see her pediatrician. On examination, she was lethargic and confused to the extent that she could not recall the current month or her own age. Her liver was enlarged, the blood aspartate and alanine aminotransferase concentrations were elevated, and she met the diagnostic criteria for Reye's syndrome.*

## CLINICAL BACKGROUND

In 1963, Reye and colleagues described in *Lancet* a syndrome characterized by acute encephalopathy associated with fatty degeneration of the liver, typically following a viral illness. Reye's syndrome is diagnosed almost exclusively in children and in its most severe forms can lead to delirium, coma, and death. In the United States, the case fatality rate from this disease ranges between about 25% and 45%.

After 3 decades of research, the cause of Reye's syndrome still is not fully understood. Several epidemiologic studies, however, have provided evidence of an association between use of aspirin during a viral illness and subsequent development of Reye's syndrome. Although the association of Reye's syndrome with aspirin use was not proved beyond doubt, health professionals acted upon the evidence provided by these studies and recommended that aspirin not be used to treat symptoms associated with viral illnesses in children. Subsequently, as the use of aspirin among children declined, so did the occurrence of Reye's syndrome. The studies that linked aspirin use with the occurrence of Reye's syndrome were based upon a case-control design. In this chapter, case-control studies are described in detail.

## INTRODUCTION

As with cohort studies, case-control investigations typically are designed to assess the association between disease occurrence and an exposure suspected of causing (or preventing) that disease. In many situations, however, a case-control study is more efficient than a cohort study because a smaller sample size is required. The key feature of a case-control study that distinguishes it from a cohort study is selection of subjects based upon their disease status. The investigator selects cases from among those persons who have the disease of interest and controls from among those who do not. In a well-designed case-control study, cases are selected from a clearly defined population, sometimes called the **source population.** The investigator then chooses controls from the same population that yielded the cases. The prior exposure histories of cases and controls are examined in order to assess relationships between exposure and disease. The basic design of a case-control study is shown in Figure 9–1.

The approach to the design of a case-control study can be illustrated by one study of the association between salicylate use and the risk of Reye's syndrome. Using a statewide surveillance system, the investigators attempted to identify all cases with Reye's syndrome in Ohio. To select controls, they identified children in the statewide community who had experienced viral illnesses similar to those reported by the cases. Parents of all subjects were interviewed and asked about their child's use of medication during the illness. Only aspirin was taken significantly more frequently by cases than by controls—93% of case children but only 66% of control children (Halpin et al, 1982). The design of this study is illustrated schematically in Figure 9–2.

This investigation illustrates several important features of case-control studies. First, the design provides an efficient means of studying rare diseases. Case-control studies tend to be more feasible than other types of epidemiologic investigations, such as cohort studies, because fewer subjects are required. The smaller sample size requirement is accompanied by a reduction in cost. Second, case-control studies allow the researcher to investigate several risk fac-

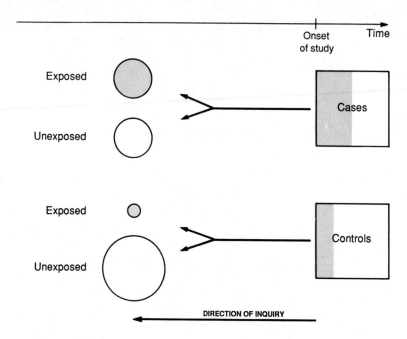

**Figure 9–1.** Schematic diagram of the design of a case-control study.

tors. In this example, the investigators evaluated several medications as possible risk factors for Reye's syndrome. Third, as with other nonexperimental or observational studies, case-control investigations do not "prove" causality, but they can provide suggestive evidence of a causal relationship that warrants public health intervention to reduce exposure to the risk factor.

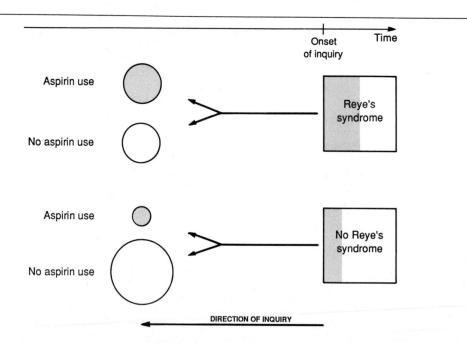

**Figure 9–2.** Schematic diagram of a case-control study of aspirin use during a viral illness among children and the subsequent risk of developing Reye's syndrome.

## DESIGN OF CASE-CONTROL STUDIES

In this section, several aspects of case-control design are discussed, including sources of cases, sources of controls, and collection of information.

### Cases

One of the first steps is to identify and select cases—a step that also determines the source population. Case identification should be complete, and the source population—ie, the population from which cases arise—should be well defined. For example, cases might be sampled at random from all patients within a geographic region, such as a state of the USA, who are diagnosed with Reye's syndrome during the study period or from all cases that occur among subscribers to a health maintenance organization. The source population in the first instance is the state and in the second instance the subscribers to the health maintenance organization. These cases may be identified by reviewing hospital records, other medical records, or death certificates, through institutional or population-based disease registries, or by means of surveillance systems.

In some situations, complete identification of cases in a well-defined source population may be too time-consuming or otherwise not possible or feasible. If so, a common alternative involves use of a "convenience sample." Cases might be sampled from those admitted to particular hospitals, or from those seen in particular clinics. Although such cases often can be identified easily, the underlying source population may not be well defined, making it difficult to generalize results.

The investigator typically studies newly diagnosed, or **incident cases,** though sometimes it is necessary to include previously existing, or **prevalent cases.** The main reason for not including prevalent cases is that the exposure may affect the prognosis or the duration of the illness. If it does, then the exposure status of existing, prevalent cases will tend to differ from that of all cases. For example, suppose that prior aspirin use either prevents death or prolongs the duration of Reye's syndrome. Prevalent cases of Reye's syndrome would then have a higher reported use of aspirin than would all cases with this disease. A case-control comparison of aspirin use would be distorted by this inflated estimate for cases. The general principle involved is that the likelihood of a case being included in the study must not depend on whether that case was exposed to the risk factor of interest.

Another important step in designing a case-control study is to specify the case definition. The criteria should minimize the likelihood that true cases are missed (ie, the criteria must be **sensitive**). At the same time, falsely classifying a nonaffected person as a case should be avoided (ie, the criteria must be **specific**). In general, there is a trade-off between the desire to include all cases (especially when the disease is extremely rare) and the desire to prevent dilution of the case group with nonaffected persons. Moreover, restrictive criteria may require information that is unavailable for some subjects, so that such subjects could not be classified fully. In practice, inclusion criteria are chosen to minimize misclassification yet retain feasibility. For example, in the previously cited study of Reye's syndrome in Ohio, cases met the criteria involving pathologic evidence of cerebral or meningeal inflammation, fatty changes in the liver, increased blood transaminase levels, and absence of other known explanations for the neurologic and hepatic processes.

### Controls

The next key step in case-control study design is to identify and select controls. Ideally, controls are chosen at random from the source population. If the source population is a state, city, or other well-defined area, controls in that area might be contacted by dialing telephone numbers at random (random-digit dialing), by visiting residences, by mailing letters soliciting participation, or by other means. An important goal is to select controls so that participation does not depend on exposure. An exposed member of the source population should be as likely to become a subject as an unexposed member. If participation does depend on exposure, then the case-control comparison may be distorted. In the previously cited study of Reye's syndrome in Ohio, the investigators attempted to select controls by first enumerating subjects in the community with a viral illness (the source population) and then selecting a control at random from the full roster of eligible children. This approach to selecting controls is unlikely to be influenced by aspirin use. Accordingly, aspirin use within this control group is likely to be comparable to that of the source population.

### Determination of Exposure

Once cases and controls are selected, information must be collected on prior exposure to the risk factor of interest as well as to other exposures. The goal is to obtain as accurate information as is possible about each individual's exposure to the main risk factors and other exposures. The information concerning other exposures is used to determine whether association of disease with a risk factor is due to the exposure of interest or to other characteristics of exposed persons. Since factors cannot affect risk after the disease occurs, the timing of exposures is critical. With slowly developing diseases that lack early evidence of involvement, establishing the temporal sequence of exposure and disease onset can be difficult or impossible.

Interviews and questionnaires are the most common means of determining a subject's exposure history. Interviews can be conducted face-to-face or by telephone. To ensure that information from cases and controls is obtained in the same manner, interviews should be standardized, monitored, and conducted by trained interviewers. Interviews are useful for collecting data because questions may cover a wide range of potential risk factors, costs are relatively low, and information can be obtained on exposures that occurred years prior to the onset of illness. On occasion, there is concern that cases and controls may report exposures differently, perhaps distorting case-control comparisons. For example, cases—perhaps in an attempt to explain their illnesses—may overreport exposures. This is of particular concern when there has been a great deal of publicity about the association between the exposure and the disease of interest.

Information concerning risk factors may be obtained also from medical, occupational, or other records. These methods of obtaining information are not based upon self-reporting and consequently should avoid the reporting bias that may occur when information is obtained by interviewing. The amount of information found in records often is limited, however, so that all of the data of interest may not be available. Furthermore, this information may not be recorded in a standardized manner, leading to variability in subject classification.

The most objective means of characterizing exposure is through the use of a biologic marker, such as measurement of an agent—or an indicator of an agent—in blood or other specimens. There are several difficulties inherent in the use of biologic markers, however. First, obtaining the specimens can involve an invasive procedure that discourages subject participation. Second, many exposures do not have known biologic markers. Third, even if a marker exists, it may be transient and thus not present when the measurement is taken. For example, salicylate levels in blood reflect recent use of aspirin but decline rapidly after exposure is stopped. Finally, the disease state may alter metabolism, thereby distorting case-control comparisons.

The type of case-control study described above, in which newly diagnosed cases and controls are sampled from a source population, is used quite commonly. It is often called a **population-based** study because cases and controls are sampled from a defined population.

## HOSPITAL-BASED
## CASE-CONTROL STUDIES

Other types of case-control studies differ from the population-based study primarily in the way the samples of cases and controls are selected. Variations include the use of prevalent rather than incident cases and sampling of controls from a readily available,

convenient group such as hospital inpatients. The **hospital-based** case-control study is used so often that it merits mention. In this type of study, the investigator typically selects cases from persons admitted with the disease of interest to a particular hospital or hospitals and controls from persons admitted with other conditions. The researcher then obtains information from cases and controls, often by interviewing them in the hospital.

The hospital-based approach can be illustrated by a case-control study of Reye's syndrome. The cases were selected from children admitted with Reye's syndrome to any of a preselected group of tertiary care hospitals. Controls were selected from children admitted to these same hospitals with an antecedent illness, presumably of viral origin. Parents were interviewed to assess prior aspirin exposure. Twenty-six of the 27 cases—but only six of the 22 hospitalized controls—had been exposed to a salicylate-containing medication. In nearly every instance, the salicylate was aspirin (Hurwitz et al, 1987).

The hospital-based case-control study can be very convenient, since cases and controls are found in the same institutions. Moreover, potential subjects, if not too ill, may be particularly willing to participate. For example, they may have more time than would normally be available. Factors such as socioeconomic status that might influence hospitalization at a particular facility tend to be balanced between cases and controls within a hospital-based case-control study.

Although they can be convenient, hospital-based studies also are susceptible to distorted results. First, cases and controls in a hospital-based study may not arise from a single, well-defined population—in contrast to the population-based case-control studies described previously. This could happen, for example, if referral patterns to particular hospitals varied across different diagnoses. Moreover, controls in a hospital-based case-control study are in a hospital because they are ill, and that condition may be associated with—even caused by—the exposure of interest. If so, then the exposure histories of controls may differ from those of the source population, and a distorted case-control comparison may result. Several selection criteria for hospital-based controls that may help to reduce this type of distortion are listed in Table 9–1.

These difficulties probably underlie a decline in popularity of hospital-based case-control studies. Despite these problems, however, hospital-based case-control studies are still performed. Typically, they are easier and quicker to conduct than population-based studies, since cases and controls are identified efficiently. As a consequence, they may be less expensive. Furthermore, the collection of exposure information from medical records and biologic markers is easier in the hospital environment. Subjects in the hospital are more accessible for interview than persons in the community. As already noted, hospital-

**Table 9–1.** Approaches to sampling of controls in hospital-based case-control studies.

Select controls from a variety of different diagnostic groups, so that no particular risk factors will be overrepresented.
Select controls from patients with acute conditions, so that earlier exposures could not have been influenced by the condition.
Do not select patients who have multiple concurrent conditions.
Do not select patients with diagnoses known to be related to the risk factor of interest.

based controls may be more cooperative with the investigators since they are ill and, for example, may want to advance medical knowledge.

Despite these differences in approaches and the subtle differences in interpretation that may result, the basic case-control design remains intact. Cases are selected from those with the disease of interest and controls from those without that disease. The relative strengths of population-based and hospital-based case-control studies are summarized in Table 9–2. In brief, the hospital-based approach offers logistical advantages, whereas the population-based approach tends to provide a clearer definition of the source population.

## SELECTION BIAS

Bias is a systematic error in a study that distorts the results and limits the validity of conclusions, as will be discussed in Chapter 10. Bias can occur for a variety of reasons, most of which can affect any type of study. One form—selection bias—poses a particular threat to case-control studies. This form of bias, as suggested by its name, reflects systematic errors that arise from the way in which subjects are selected. If selection of cases, controls, or both is influenced by prior exposure, this bias may be present. In particular, if the exposure of the cases studied differs from that of all cases arising from the source population— or if exposure of controls differs from that of persons

in the source population without the disease— selection bias may be present.

The development of selection bias is illustrated schematically in Figure 9–3. The shaded figures represent persons who were exposed and the unshaded figures those who were not. In the source population, one-third of persons with disease were exposed. Among the cases included in the study, however, two-thirds were exposed. That is to say, exposed persons with disease were more likely than unexposed persons with disease to be selected for study. In this illustration, an opposite sampling pattern is displayed for persons without disease. In this group, exposed persons were less likely to be selected for study than were unexposed persons. Obviously, comparison of exposure histories of sampled cases and controls in this study would yield a result different from that achieved by contrasting exposure histories of persons with and without disease in the source population.

There are at least three ways in which this type of bias could arise in case-control studies of Reye's syndrome:

**(1)** Preferential diagnosis of exposed cases may lead to selection bias. After the initial publicity concerning the suspected association of Reye's syndrome with aspirin use, physicians may have been more inclined to suspect the diagnosis of Reye's syndrome among children who were known to have used aspirin for a preceding viral illness. If so, children with Reye's syndrome who did not take aspirin could have been underrepresented within the case group, creating selection bias.

**(2)** Low participation may lead to selection bias. For example, parents of eligible subjects may refuse

**Table 9–2.** Relative strengths of population-based and hospital-based case-control studies.

| Population-Based | Hospital-Based |
|---|---|
| Source population is better defined | Subjects are more accessible |
| Easier to make certain that cases and controls derive from the same source population | Subjects tend to be more cooperative |
| | Background characteristics of cases and controls may be balanced |
| Exposure histories of controls more likely to reflect those of persons without the disease of interest | Easier to collect exposure information from medical records and biologic specimens |

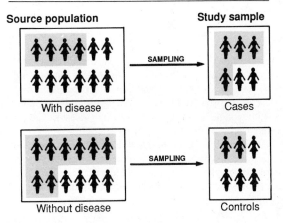

**Figure 9–3.** Schematic diagram of the origin of selection bias in a case-control study. The shaded figures represent persons who were exposed and the unshaded figures indicate persons who were unexposed.

to participate, or physicians may advise their patients not to participate. If aspirin use of those who did not participate differed from that of those who are enrolled, selection bias must be suspected.

(3) Errors in sampling controls from the source population can also create selection bias. For example, if sampled controls had conditions that would make them more or less likely to use aspirin than other children, selection bias could occur.

These examples illustrate some of the many ways in which selection bias can arise in case-control studies. The particular susceptibility of case-control studies to selection bias reflects the need to obtain two samples: a sample of cases and a sample of controls. Unless each sample is obtained without regard to exposure, results may be biased.

## MATCHING

**Confounding,** as will be discussed in detail in Chapter 10, is a distortion of results that occurs when the apparent effects of the exposure of interest actually are attributable entirely or in part to the effects of an extraneous variable. Confounding is likely to occur when persons exposed to the risk factor of interest differ from the nonexposed with respect to the prevalence of other risk factors.

There are several possible approaches to the control of confounding, including matched sampling, as described here. **Matching** is a popular approach to the control of confounding in case-control studies. Its popularity reflects the sense that matching cases and controls forces these groups to be similar with respect to important risk factors and thereby makes case-control comparisons less subject to confounding. This perception about matching is true provided one conducts the appropriate matched analysis.

The first step in matching is to identify a case. One or more potential controls with the same values for each matching factor as the case are then selected from the source population. The process of matching by race and gender is illustrated schematically in Figure 9–4. In order to match on a continuous variable, such as age, it is typically necessary to form categories, such as 5-year intervals (years 10–14, 15–19, 20–24, . . .). In a study with matching on age in 5-year intervals, for example, a 17-year-old black female case would be matched to a black female control aged 15–19 from the source population. As in an unmatched study, these controls come from the defined source population. More than one control can be matched to each case, but the ratio of controls to cases rarely exceeds 4:1, because additional controls beyond this ratio add relatively little to the statistical power of the study.

The use of matching is common in clinical studies,

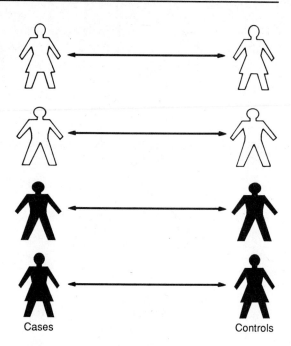

Cases          Controls

**Figure 9–4.** Schematic diagram of the process of matching controls to cases by race and gender.

especially when the disease of interest is extremely rare. In this situation, there are a small number of potential cases and a large number of potential controls. Matching can increase the statistical efficiency of case-control comparisons and thus achieve a specified level of statistical power with a smaller sample size. The matching protocol often simplifies decisions about how to sample controls. In addition, matching tends to ensure that case-control differences in the risk factor of interest cannot be explained by reference to the matched variables.

These advantages of matching must be weighed against a number of disadvantages, however. As indicated in Table 9–3, matching can be time-consuming and therefore expensive. Any potential cases or controls that cannot be matched must be discarded, which can be viewed as a wasteful process. Any variable that is matched in a study cannot be evaluated as a risk factor in that investigation. Finally, matching on ordinal or continuous variables may result in categories that are too broad to completely remove the effects of the matched variables from the exposure-disease relationship.

## ANALYSIS

The type of analysis employed in a case-control study depends upon whether subjects were sampled in an unmatched or in a matched approach. These two analytic strategies are described in the following sections.

**Table 9–3.** Advantages and disadvantages of matching in case-control studies.

**Advantages**

May increase the precision of case-control comparisons and thus allow a smaller study

The sampling process is easy to understand and explain

If analyzed correctly, provides reassurance that matched variables cannot explain case-control differences in the risk factor of interest

**Disadvantages**

May be time-consuming and expensive to perform

Some potential cases and controls may be excluded because matches cannot be made

The matched variables cannot be evaluated as risk factors in the study population

For continuous or ordinal variables, matching categories may be too broad, and residual case-control differences in these variables may persist

## Unmatched Design

The data obtained in an unmatched case-control study can be summarized as indicated in Table 9–4. For simplicity, only two levels of exposure are discussed here, though the basic methods can be expanded to include multiple levels of exposure. Each subject can be classified into one of the four basic groups defined by disease and prior exposure status:

A. Cases who were exposed
B. Cases who were not exposed
C. Controls who were exposed
D. Controls who were not exposed

The format of Table 9–4 should appear familiar, since it resembles that of Table 8–6. Although the summary tables for cohort and case-control studies are similar, it is important to remember that the underlying approaches to sampling differ, and the analysis must account for these differences. In a cohort study, sampling is based upon exposure status, and the investigator thus determines the total numbers of exposed $(A + C)$ and unexposed subjects $(B + D)$ that are included in the study. Risk of disease development then can be estimated separately for exposed and unexposed groups, and these two risks can be compared in a risk ratio $(RR)$.

A case-control study, on the other hand, begins with sampling of persons with and without the disease of interest $(A + B$ and $C + D$, respectively). With this approach, the proportion of persons in the study who have the disease is no longer determined by the disease risk in the source population but rather by the choice of the investigator. That is, a disease that occurs infrequently in the source population can be oversampled, so that affected individuals constitute a large proportion of the study sample. This ability to oversample affected individuals is why case-control studies are statistically efficient for the study of rare diseases.

Once the investigator determines the ratio of persons with and without the disease of interest in a case-control study, risk of disease no longer can be estimated. As shown in the following section, however, an indirect estimate of the incidence rate ratio can still be obtained in a case-control study.

## Odds Ratio

With the notation introduced in Table 9–4, the probability that a case was exposed previously is estimated by:

$$\text{Case exposure probability} = \frac{\textbf{Exposed cases}}{\textbf{All cases}}$$

$$= \frac{A}{A + B}$$

The odds of exposure for cases represent the probability that a case was exposed divided by the probability that a case was not exposed. The odds then are estimated by:

**Odds of case exposure**

$$= \frac{\textbf{Exposed cases}}{\textbf{All cases}} \Big/ \frac{\textbf{Unexposed cases}}{\textbf{All cases}}$$

$$= \frac{A}{A + B} \Big/ \frac{B}{A + B} = \frac{A}{B}$$

Similarly, the odds of exposure among controls are estimated by:

$$\text{Odds of control exposure} = \frac{C}{D}$$

The odds of exposure for cases divided by the odds of exposure for controls are expressed as the **odds ratio** (**OR**). Substituting from the preceding equations, the OR is estimated by:

$$\text{Odds ratio} = \frac{\textbf{Odds of case exposure}}{\textbf{Odds of control exposure}}$$

$$= \frac{A}{B} \Big/ \frac{C}{D} = \frac{A \times D}{B \times C}$$

The $OR$ is sometimes termed the exposure odds ratio or the cross-product of Table 9–4, because it results from dividing the product of entries on one diagonal of this table by the product of entries on the cross-diagonal.

**Table 9–4.** Summary of data collected in an unmatched case-control study.

|  | Exposed | Unexposed | Total |
|---|---|---|---|
| Cases | $A$ | $B$ | $A + B$ |
| Controls | $C$ | $D$ | $C + D$ |
| Total | $A + C$ | $B + D$ | $A + B + C + D$ |

**Table 9–5.** Summary of data from a hypothetical unmatched case-control study of Reye's syndrome and aspirin use.

|  | Aspirin Use | No Aspirin Use | Total |
|---|---|---|---|
| Cases | 190 | 10 | 200 |
| Controls | 130 | 70 | 200 |
| Total | 320 | 80 | 400 |

When incident cases and controls are sampled from the same source population (with selection independent of prior exposure), the exposure *OR* provides a valid estimate of the incidence rate ratio. In other words, if properly designed, a case-control study can yield a measure of association between exposure and disease that approximates the incidence rate ratio.

The calculation of the *OR* can be illustrated by data from a hypothetical case-control study of aspirin use and Reye's syndrome. The findings of this hypothetical investigation are summarized in Table 9–5. The *OR* for these data is as follows:

$$\text{Odds ratio} = \frac{A \times D}{B \times C} = \frac{190 \times 70}{10 \times 130} = 10.2$$

In other words, the odds of aspirin use for patients with Reye's syndrome were almost seven times greater than the odds for aspirin use among controls in this study. To the extent that the *OR* provides a valid estimate of the incidence rate ratio, one could conclude from this investigation that use of aspirin for a preceding viral illness increased the likelihood of developing Reye's syndrome sevenfold.

As with the risk ratio, a 95% confidence interval around the point estimate of the *OR* can be calculated. A formula for calculating an approximate 95% confidence interval is given in Appendix D. With the data presented in Table 9–5, the approximate 95% confidence interval for the *OR* is 5.1 to 20.5. That is, the data from this hypothetical study are consistent with a strong to a very strong positive association between the use of aspirin and the development of Reye's syndrome. This association is highly unlikely to have occurred by chance alone, since the null value of the *OR* (null value = 1) is far outside of the 95% confidence interval. The point estimate and confience interval for this odds ratio are illustrated in Figure 9–5.

## Matched Design

In a matched case-control study, the analysis must account for the matched sampling scheme. When one control is matched to each case, the summary data can be presented in the format shown in Table 9–6. An extension of this basic format can be employed for situations in which ratio of controls to cases differs from 1:1. Although there are four cells in Table 9–6, the entries into this format are quite different from what we find in previous tables. Each entry into Table 9–6 represents not one subject but two (a matched case-control pair). That is, each case-control pair can be classified into one of the four basic combinations of exposure status:

W. Both case and control exposed
X. Case exposed, but control unexposed
Y. Case unexposed, but control exposed
Z. Both case and control unexposed

Case-control pairs that are entered into cells *W* and *Z* are referred to as **concordant pairs,** because the exposure statuses of cases and controls in these pairs are the same. Case-control pairs that are entered into cells *X* and *Y,* in contrast, are referred to as **discordant pairs,** since the exposure statuses of cases and controls in these pairs are different.

The *OR* for a pair-matched case-control study is given by a simple ratio:

$$\text{Odds ratio} = \frac{X}{Y}$$

This odds ratio can be interpreted in the same manner as the *OR* for unmatched studies.

To illustrate the calculation of the *OR* from a matched study, the results of a hypothetical case-control study with 200 matched case-control pairs are shown in Table 9–7. The *OR* from this study is as follows:

$$\text{Odds ratio} = \frac{X}{Y} = \frac{57}{5} = 11.4$$

A 95% confidence interval around the point estimate of the matched *OR* can be calculated. A formula for calculating an approximate 95% confidence interval is given in Appendix D. With the data presented in

**Table 9–6.** Summary data format for a matched case-control study with one control per case.

|  | Control Exposed | Control Unexposed | Total |
|---|---|---|---|
| Case exposed | W | X | W + X |
| Case unexposed | Y | Z | Y + Z |
| Total | W + Y | X + Z | W + X + Y + Z |

**Table 9–7.** Summary data from a hypothetical matched case-control study of aspirin use and risk of Reye's syndrome.

|  | Control Exposed | Control Unexposed | Total |
|---|---|---|---|
| Case exposed | 132 | 57 | 189 |
| Case unexposed | 5 | 6 | 11 |
| Total | 137 | 63 | 200 |

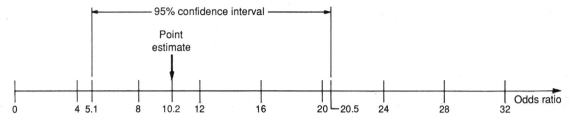

**Figure 9–5.** Point estimate and 95% confidence interval for odds ratio comparing aspirin use among patients with Reye's syndrome and controls.

Table 9–7, the approximate 95% confidence interval for the *OR* is 4.6 to 28.3. That is, the data from the hypothetical matched case-control study are consistent with a strong to a very strong positive association between the use of aspirin and the development of Reye's syndrome. This association is highly unlikely to have occurred by chance, since the null value of the *OR* (null value = 1) is far outside the 95% confidence interval.

## SUMMARY

In this chapter, the basic approach to the design and analysis of case-control studies was presented, with illustrations drawn from the literature on the relationship between aspirin use and the risk of Reye's syndrome. A case-control study is a type of observational investigation in which subjects are enrolled on the basis of the presence or absence of a particular disease (eg, Reye's syndrome) and then evaluated to determine their history of exposure to risk factors of interest (eg, aspirin use for viral illness).

The advantages and disadvantages of the case-control approach are summarized in Table 9–8. The advantages of this design are chiefly logistical. In particular, rare diseases (Reye's syndrome is one example) and those with long latency periods can be studied efficiently. The sample size required for a case-control study tends to be smaller than would be needed for an alternative design, such as a cohort study. As a result, the expense of conducting a case-control study may be substantially less than the cost of a cohort study. Furthermore, reliance on historical information allows rapid completion of a case-control study. The ability to reach a prompt conclusion is particularly important if the disease is potentially life-threatening, as is Reye's syndrome, because future cases might be prevented by authoritative action to limit exposure to a suspected risk factor.

The disadvantages of case-control studies relate primarily to their susceptibility to systematic errors. Since cases and controls are sampled separately, it is possible that these groups may not arise from the same source population. Bias can be introduced into the study results if exposure status is associated with the likelihood of including cases or controls into the study. Reliance upon subject recall of earlier exposures or the use of historical records can lead to imprecise or inaccurate classification of exposure.

The decision to conduct a case-control study typically is motivated by a desire to explore the relationship between a specific risk factor and a particular disease. Ideally, the cases and the controls should derive from a single well-defined source population, such as a state (a **population-based** sampling scheme). An attempt may be made to identify all newly diagnosed cases (**incident cases**) within the source population, particularly when the disease is rare or the source population is modest in size. Cases may be identified from hospital records, surveillance systems, death certificates, or other sources. Careful criteria for the presence of disease must be established in order to minimize false inclusions or exclusions.

Controls typically are sampled from the population that gave rise to the cases. Occasionally, for purposes of convenience, **hospital-based samples** of cases and controls are selected. The hospital-based approach tends to have the advantages of accessibility to the subjects and cooperative study participants. On the other hand, cases and controls may derive from dissimilar source populations in a hospital-based study, and exposure status might influence the likelihood of inclusion in this type of investigation.

**Matching** of controls to cases on the basis of known risk factors for the disease of interest is a common practice in case-control studies. The intent of matching is usually to decrease the possibility of **confounding,** or mixing of the effect of interest with the effects of other risk factors. Matching can increase the statistical precision of estimates and thereby allow a smaller sample size. On the other hand, matching can be time-consuming and wasteful of information from subjects who are not successfully matched and for that reason must be discarded.

The process of subject selection in a case-control study precludes the estimation of risks (or rates), and the risk ratio therefore cannot be calculated directly from case-control data. An indirect estimate of the risk ratio, however, can be calculated in a case-control study. This measure is referred to as the **odds**

**Table 9–8.** Advantages and disadvantages of case-control studies.

**Advantages**
Efficient for the study of rare diseases
Efficient for the study of chronic diseases
Tend to require a smaller sample size than other designs
Less expensive than alternative designs
May be completed more rapidly than alternative designs
**Disadvantages**
Risk of disease cannot be estimated directly
Not efficient for the study of rare exposures
More susceptible to selection bias than alternative designs
Information on exposure may be less accurate than that
    available in alternative designs

ratio and is defined as the odds of exposure among cases divided by the odds of exposure among controls. The approach to calculating the odds ratio depends upon whether subjects were sampled in an unmatched or matched fashion. In either instance, a point estimate and 95% confidence interval for the odds ratio can be calculated as a measure of association between exposure and disease occurrence.

A number of case-control studies of Reye's syndrome were conducted. Cases and controls were sampled using a variety of different approaches in these studies. The most consistent risk factor that emerged from these studies—other than young age and the presence of a preceding viral illness—was the use of aspirin. The strength of the association between aspirin and Reye's syndrome and the consistency of results across studies suggested that this was a cause-and-effect relationship. The decline in the incidence of Reye's syndrome with decreasing use of aspirin to treat viral illnesses in children further supported this explanation.

## STUDY QUESTIONS

**Directions:** For each question, select the single best answer.

**Questions 1–3:** In an unmatched case-control study of risk factors for congenital defects of the neural tube, maternal deficiency of folate was found in 15 of 100 mothers of cases and 10 of 200 mothers of controls:

1. The odds of exposure among cases is:
   A. 15/100
   B. (15/100)/(85/100)
   C. (15/100)/(10/200)
   D. (15 × 190)/(85 × 10)
   E. (85 × 10)/(15 × 190)
2. The odds ratio for exposure is:
   A. 15/100
   B. (15/100)/(85/100)
   C. (15/100)/(10/200)
   D. (15 × 190)/(85 × 10)
   E. (85 × 10)/(15 × 190)

**Questions 3–4:** In a case-control study of risk factors for migraine headaches, the odds ratio for high levels of daily stress was 3.2 with a 95% confidence interval of 1.7 to 6.1.

3. Based upon these data, the minimal percentage increase in the odds of high levels of daily stress for cases compared to controls at a 95% level of confidence was:
   A. 1.7%
   B. 6.1%
   C. 17%
   D. 61%
   E. 70%

4. If the sample size is doubled, the width of the 95% confidence intervals is expected to:
   A. Decrease
   B. Increase
   C. Remain unchanged
   D. Include the null value
   E. Change, but the direction cannot be predicted

**Questions 5–6:** In a case-control study of risk factors for oral cancer, the odds ratio for consumption of fresh fruits is 0.6 with a 95% confidence interval of 0.4 to 0.9.

5. Based upon these data, the effect of fresh fruit upon the risk of oral cancer is:
   A. Protective
   B. No effect
   C. Harmful
   D. Uncertain from the information presented

6. At the 5% level of statistical significance, the association between fresh vegetable consumption and risk of oral cancer is:
   A. Statistically significant
   B. Not statistically significant
   C. Of uncertain statistical significance without a hypothesis test
   D. Not appropriately assessed by statistical significance because randomization was not performed

7. Each of the following is likely to be an advantage of case-control studies as opposed to prospective cohort studies EXCEPT
   A. Less expensive
   B. Can be completed more rapidly
   C. More efficient for the study of rare diseases
   D. More efficient for the study of diseases that develop slowly
   E. The temporal relationship between exposure and disease is better refined

8. In a case-control study of exercise as a protective factor against the development of osteoporosis, cases tend to overestimate their level of exercise

more than controls. The likely effect on the observed association is:

A. To increase the apparent protection
B. To decrease the apparent protection
C. None
D. Impossible to predict from the information given

9. In a case-control study of risk factors for ectopic pregnancies, the use of an intrauterine device (IUD) was more common among cases than controls. The strength of association increased with longer duration of use of an IUD. This is an example of:

A. Latency
B. Confounding
C. Dose-response
D. Misclassification
E. A cohort effect

10. In a case-control study of diabetes mellitus as a risk factor in the development of chronic renal disease, the odds ratio was 3.0 and the results were statistically significant at the 5% level. This means that:

A. Five percent of patients with chronic renal disease had diabetes mellitus
B. Five percent of patients with diabetes mellitus developed chronic renal failure
C. Five percent more patients with chronic renal failure had a history of diabetes mellitus than controls
D. If there was an association between diabetes and renal disease, there is a 5% possibility that the association occurred by chance alone

## FURTHER READING

Greenberg RS, Ibrahim MA: The case-control study. In: *Oxford Textbook of Public Health,* 2nd ed. Vol 2. Holland WW, Detels R, Knox G (editors). Oxford Univ Press, 1991.

## REFERENCES

CDC: Reye syndrome surveillance—United States, 1989. MMWR 1991;40:88.

Daniels SR, Greenberg RS, Ibrahim MA. Scientific uncertainties in the studies of salicylate use and Reye's syndrome. JAMA 1983;249:1311.

Halpin TJ et al: Reye's syndrome and medication use. JAMA 1982;248:687.

Hurwitz ES et al: Public Health Service study of Reye's syndrome and medications. JAMA 1987;257:1905.

Reye RDK, Morgan G, Baral J: Encephalopathy and fatty degeneration of the viscera: A disease entity in childhood. Lancet 1963;2:749.

# 10

## PATIENT PROFILE

*A 45-year-old man began working as a production supervisor and his employer required that he undergo a complete medical examination. His physician learned that the patient's father had died of myocardial infarction at age 65. On physical examination, the patient was moderately obese and his blood pressure was 140/86. The remainder of the examination revealed no notable abnormalities. The patient's total serum cholesterol level (nonfasting) was 242 mg/dL.*

*According to the National Cholesterol Education Program (NCEP) guidelines, a total serum cholesterol concentration greater than 240 mg/dL is an indication for possible pharmacologic lowering of serum cholesterol. A value of 200–239 mg/dL is considered borderline and should trigger dietary intervention, and a value less than 200 mg/dL is considered normal.*

*Based on the initial cholesterol results, the physician asked the patient to return in 2 weeks for further testing. On repeat measurement, the total serum cholesterol was 198 mg/dL on a fasting lipid profile. Table 10–1 lists several different factors that could explain the observed variability in measured total serum cholesterol. The source of this variability in the measured total cholesterol level had important implications for how the physician treated this patient.*

## VARIABILITY IN MEDICAL RESEARCH

Difficulties in the interpretation of test results of individual patients are magnified when groups of patients are studied. The sources of variability in test results and errors in medical research are discussed in this chapter. Appreciation of these issues is important for the interpretation and appropriate application of research findings in the clinical setting.

Variability in measurements can be either random or systematic. A schematic representation of random and systematic variation is shown in Figure 10–1. The shots at the targets in both A and B are centered around the middle, but in A the shots are less scattered and have less variability, or more **precision.** In targets C and D the scatter is similar, but in target D the cluster of shots is off center. This might occur, for example, if the sight of the gun was bent. The precision is comparable, but the result in D is systematically off target or **biased.** The results in target C are accurate, or valid. It is important to consider the accuracy and precision of any measurements made in the medical setting. Variability can occur at a number of different levels (eg, individual, population) in clinical medicine and medical research (Table 10–1). The variability inherent in the method of measurement is important at each level.

## Variability Within the Individual

The first level of concern is variability in the true value of a person's characteristics over time. This was a source of concern for the clinician in the Patient Profile. Some potential sources of individual variability are listed in Table 10–2. The source of this variation can be the individual being measured, the instrument being used to perform the measurement, the technician taking the measurement, or the person interpreting the result. Variation can occur because of biologic changes in an individual over time. These changes may occur on a minute-to-minute basis (eg, heart rate), follow a regular diurnal pattern (eg, body temperature), or progress with normal development (eg, height or weight).

When the variation within a subject is large, a single measurement may not adequately represent the "true" status of that individual. By repeating a test, the physician may obtain a better understanding of the true value and its variability. This may also give the clinician a clue about variability or error due to the measurement technique. In the Patient Profile, different results were obtained when the total serum cholesterol was measured a second time, when the patient was fasting. It is unlikely, however, that the fasting state alone could cause such a drop in total serum cholesterol. Furthermore, it is unlikely that the patient could have made the kind of dietary or other alterations in 2 weeks that would lead to the observed change in total serum cholesterol.

**Table 10–1.** Levels of variability.

**Individual**
Individual variability
Measurement variability
**Population**
Genetic variability between individuals
Environmental variability
Measurement variability
**Sample**
Manner of sampling
Size of sample
Measurement variability

**Table 10–2.** Potential sources of variability in measurements of individuals.

**Individual characteristics**
Diurnal variation
Changes related to factors such as age, diet, and exercise
environmental factors such as season or temperature
**Measurement characteristics**
Poor calibration of the instrument
Inherent lack of precision of the instrument
Misreading or misrecording information from the instrument
by the technician

## Variability Related to Measurement

Laboratory measurements of total serum cholesterol are notorious for both variability and error. In order to determine which value—198 mg/dL or 242 mg/dL—was closer to the truth, the physician in the Patient Profile would need to know whether or not both measurements were obtained in the same laboratory. For example, the first result may have been obtained from a desktop analyzer in the physician's office, while the lipid profile may have been measured in a standardized laboratory. In reality, the physician may not be able to discern readily which value is closer to the truth. This is one reason that programs with guidelines that support cutoff points for clinical decision making, such as the NCEP, often recommend that elevated values be confirmed by repeated measurements over time before treatment is instituted.

## Variations Within Populations

Just as there is variation in individuals, there is also variability in populations (see Table 10–2), which can be thought of as the cumulative variability of individuals. Since populations are made up of individuals with different genetic constitutions who are subject to different environmental influences, populations often exhibit more variation than individuals. Physicians use knowledge about variability in populations to define what is "normal" and "abnormal." The physician in the Patient Profile could refer to population survey data to learn that for 45-year-old males a total serum cholesterol value of 200 mg/dL is close to the 50th percentile and a value of 240 mg/dL is equivalent to the 75th percentile. Accordingly, the patient falls generally in the upper half of the population distribution of total serum cholesterol values. Assuming that the measurement is correct, this could be a result of genetic factors, environmental factors, or both.

## Variability in Research Studies

It is worthwhile asking how the clinician would know that a total serum cholesterol value in the upper end of the population distribution is disadvantageous. Are these values really unhealthy? Answers may be found in studies that have linked the level of total serum cholesterol with an increased risk of cardiovascular mortality. In cohort studies, such as the Framingham Heart Study, groups of subjects with different levels of total serum cholesterol and their subsequent experience of death from myocardial infarction or stroke were followed and compared. In these investigations, a higher level of total serum cholesterol was associated with an increased risk of death from cardiovascular disease.

When investigators perform such studies, they cannot usually study the entire population. Instead they study subsets or samples of the population. This introduces another source of variability—termed sampling variability—that is important in medical research. Using a single sample of subjects to represent the population is analogous to using a single measurement to characterize an individual. Repeated samples from the population would give different estimates of

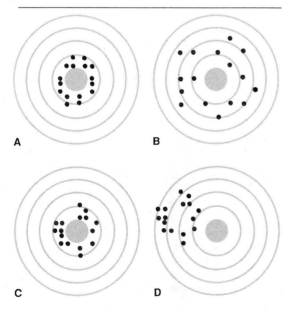

**Figure 10–1.** Schematic illustrations of increased random error (target B versus target A) and systematic error (target D versus target C).

the true population values. Sampling variability is illustrated in Figure 10–2. In the source population of 20 persons, there are five individuals (25%) with total serum cholesterol values above 240 mg/dL. In the three different samples of five subjects drawn from the source population by chance, the proportion of individuals with total serum cholesterol values above 240 mg/dL ranges from 0 to 40%. Each of these small samples presents a different picture of the source population. A larger sample size would result in less variability and would be more likely to be representative of the source population.

Variability can be important in other ways when two groups are to be compared in a study. The goal of such studies often is to determine whether there is a measurable difference between the groups. When a research paper reports no statistically significant difference between the groups, the reader must ask, Was there no difference between the two treatments in truth, or was the estimate of effect so imprecise that the investigator could not distinguish differences between the two groups (type II error)?

A graphic display of the results of two hypothetical studies of the same question is presented in Figure 10–3. In each study the investigators attempted to determine whether a cholesterol-lowering drug had a favorable effect on the risk of myocardial infarction. The effect measure that was estimated in each study

was the risk ratio. Each study compared a group of patients who were randomly allocated to receive the cholesterol-lowering drug with a group chosen to receive dietary modification alone. The researchers reached different conclusions. In the study with the smaller sample, the report indicated that the drug had no beneficial effect on risk of myocardial infarction when compared with diet therapy. In the study with the larger sample, the investigators concluded that the drug decreased the risk of myocardial infarction when compared with dietary management.

As shown in Figure 10–3, Study A had a small sample size, which resulted in imprecise estimates (ie, wide confidence intervals) of the risk of myocardial infarction in the two groups. Consequently, the two estimates overlapped, and the statistical test was not capable of distinguishing between the effects of the two treatments. The investigators concluded that there was no difference in risk of myocardial infarction between patients who received the cholesterol-lowering drug and those who received dietary therapy. In Study B, the investigator used a larger sample size yielding the same point estimates of risk in the two groups but with much more precision (ie, narrower confidence intervals) in the estimate of the effects of the drug. With this gain in precision, the statistical test was able to distinguish between the two groups and the investigator was able to infer correctly that the cholesterol-lowering drug was superior to dietary therapy.

Generally, the larger the sample size, the more precise the estimate of effect and the smaller the detectable differences between groups. In studies with very large sample sizes, small differences between groups may be judged to be statistically significant but have little biologic or clinical meaning. For example, a study of 20,000 subjects might have concluded that a 1% difference in risk of myocardial infarction was statistically significant. It is unlikely, however, that a difference in risk this small would justify prolonged use of the cholesterol-lowering agent.

## VALIDITY

*The concept of validity concerns the degree to which a measurement or study reaches a correct conclusion.* A measurement or study may lead to an incorrect (invalid) conclusion because of the effects of **bias.** The variability seen with bias is systematic or nonrandom and distorts the estimated effect. In Figure 10–1, the amount of bias can be determined by the degree to which the shots are off target in D. Unfortunately, in medical research the truth (bulls-eye) may not be known or there may no "gold standard" for comparison. As a consequence, the degree of bias often is difficult to determine.

Two different types of validity, internal validity and external validity, will be described in this chapter.

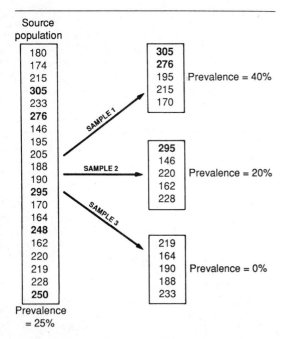

**Figure 10–2.** Schematic diagram of sampling variability. The source population of 20 persons has a 25% prevalence of hypercholesterolemia (elevated cholesterol values are presented in bold). Each of three random samples of five persons yields prevalence estimates ranging from 0 to 40%.

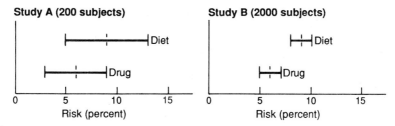

**Figure 10–3.** The effect of sample size on precision of risk estimates. Point estimates are shown as dashed vertical lines and 95% confidence intervals are shown as solid horizontal lines. In both studies, the 5-year risk of myocardial infarction was 9% among persons receiving dietary therapy and 6% among persons treated with a cholesterol-lowering drug. In the larger study, however, the 95% confidence intervals are narrower and the difference in risk between treatment groups is statistically significant.

## Internal Validity

*Internal validity is the extent to which the results of an investigation accurately reflect the true situation of the study population.* If the results are not valid in the study population, then there is little reason to suspect that they will apply to other populations. Internal validity is defined by the boundaries of the study itself. Therefore, a study is internally valid if it provides a true estimate of effect given the limits of the population studied. Measures that can be used to improve internal validity often involve restricting the type of subjects and the environment in which the study is performed. These measures decrease the impact of factors extraneous to the question of interest.

## External Validity

A result obtained in a tightly controlled environment, however, may not be applicable to more general situations. *External validity is the extent to which the results of a study are applicable to other populations.* It addresses the question, Do these results apply to other patients, such as patients who are older, sicker, or less economically advantaged than the subjects in the study? External validity often is of particular interest to clinicians who must decide if a research finding is applicable to their own clinical practice. Determining whether the results of a study can be generalized involves a judgment regarding (1) the type of subjects included in the investigation, (2) the type of patients seen by the clinician, and (3) whether there are clinically meaningful differences between the study population and other populations.

An example of problems with the generalization of study results is the criticism that too many clinical studies focus on white males. One such study is the Lipid Research Clinics-Primary Prevention Trial, which demonstrated a significant reduction in cardiovascular mortality for hypercholesterolemic white men aged 35–59 years who were placed on a cholesterol-lowering diet and medication. Do the results also apply to men of different ages with or without lower, but still abnormal, cholesterol levels and to

women? This question has led to the suggestion that federally funded research should include women and minorities in their study populations.

## Bias

*Bias is a systematic error in a study that leads to a distortion of the results.* Bias, a threat to validity, can be present in any research, but it is of particular concern in observational studies because the lack of randomization increases the chance that study groups will differ with respect to important characteristics. Bias often is subdivided into different categories based upon how it enters the study. The most common classification divides bias into three categories: selection bias, information bias, and confounding. Although these categories overlap, this classification is useful because it provides the reader with a systematic approach to evaluating bias. It should be remembered that, with the exception of confounding, which can be quantitated, the evaluation of bias is subjective and involves a judgment regarding the likelihood of its presence and the direction and potential magnitude of its effect on the results. Even though the magnitude of bias cannot be quantified, often one can infer how such a bias might influence the results of a study. It is important to discern whether the suspected bias is likely to make an association appear stronger or weaker than it really is. Overestimation of a risk ratio for a protective exposure and a separate hazardous exposure is demonstrated schematically in Figure 10–4. Underestimation of a risk ratio for a protective exposure and a hazardous exposure is shown in Figure 10–5.

## Selection Bias

A variety of procedures can be used to select subjects for a study. Usually, it is not possible to include all individuals with a particular disease or exposure in a study, so a sample of subjects must be chosen. The procedures used for the selection of subjects depend on a number of factors, including the design of the investigation, the setting of the study, and the disease and exposure of interest. Often subjects are selected in a manner that is convenient for the investigator.

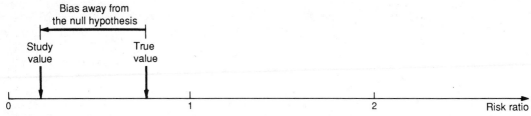

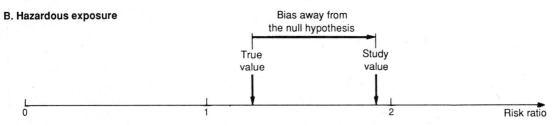

**Figure 10–4.** Overestimation of a risk ratio for (A) a protective exposure and (B) a hazardous exposure.

Under optimal circumstances, the method for inclusion of subjects leads to a valid comparison that yields correct information regarding a disease process or treatment. The selection process itself, however, may increase or decrease the chance that a relationship between the exposure and disease of interest will be detected. A schematic diagram of the steps involved in recruiting and maintaining a study population is shown in Figure 10–6. From this diagram, it is easy to see that selection factors could lead to biased results at several different steps in the process.

Some aspects of the selection of subjects lead pri-marily to problems with the generalization (extrapolation) of the results (ie, external validity). Subjects must agree to participate in a study, and this causes one of the most common problems. Volunteers for a study may differ from individuals who do not volunteer in a variety of characteristics, such as age, race, economic status, education level, and gender. Moreover, volunteers may be healthier than those who decline to participate. A study of a population limited to individuals who are employed may also make generalization of study results difficult, since people who work are generally healthier than those who do not. A

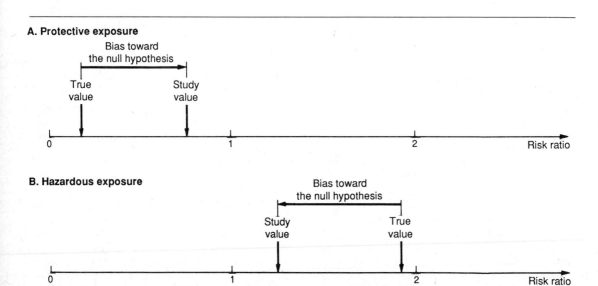

**Figure 10–5.** Underestimation of a risk ratio for (A) a protective exposure and (B) a hazardous exposure.

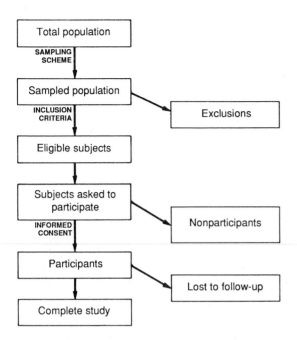

**Figure 10–6.** Steps in the selection and maintenance of subjects in a study.

comparison of health outcomes between workers and the general population may show that the workers have a more favorable outcome simply because they are healthy enough to be employed (the "healthy worker" effect).

Referral of patients to clinical facilities also can lead to distorted study conclusions. Selective referral patterns can be seen in the study of children with febrile seizures. Febrile seizures are brief, generalized seizures that occur in conjunction with temperature elevation in children aged 6 months to 6 years. There is some disagreement about whether these febrile convulsions are predictive of future seizures and other unfavorable neurologic sequelae. Ellenberg and Nelson (1980) compared the results of a number of studies on the long-term outcome of patients with febrile seizures. Studies of geographically defined populations in which affected children were followed, regardless of whether or not medical care was sought, consistently revealed a relatively low rate of unfavorable sequelae. Clinic-based studies tended to report a high frequency of adverse outcomes. Accordingly, it was concluded that clinic-based studies selectively included children at the more severe end of the clinical spectrum. The inferences that one might draw regarding the prognosis of a child with febrile seizures might be very different based upon whether a clinic-based or population-based sample was studied.

Other aspects of the selection process can diminish internal validity. *In a clinical trial or cohort study, the major potential selection bias is loss to follow-up.*

Once subjects are enrolled in the study, they may decide to discontinue participation. Certain types of subjects are more likely than others to drop out of a study. Furthermore, some subjects may die from causes other than the outcome of interest during the course of the study. At first glance, these losses may not appear to be related to selection because the subject was enrolled already in the study. If the lost subjects differ in their risk of the outcome of interest, however, biased estimates of risk may be obtained.

If the unrecognized early manifestations of the disease of interest cause exposed persons to leave the study more or less frequently than unexposed persons, a distorted conclusion might be reached. For example, in a randomized controlled trial of the effects of a cholesterol-lowering drug versus diet on prevention of myocardial infarctions, bias might be introduced if drug-treated patients with coronary insufficiency were more likely to develop side effects from treatment and withdrew from participation, whereas patients with coronary insufficiency receiving dietary therapy remained in the study.

Selection bias is of particular importance in case-control studies (see Chapter 9) where the investigator must select two study groups, cases and controls, in a setting in which the exposure has already occurred. For example, it must be decided whether to use existing (prevalent) cases who are available at the time of study regardless of the duration of their disease or limit eligibility to newly diagnosed (incident) cases. If the risk factor of interest also is a prognostic factor, the use of prevalent cases can lead to a biased conclusion. Consider, for example, a case-control study of total serum cholesterol as a risk factor for myocardial infarction. Suppose that myocardial infarction patients with very high total serum cholesterol levels are more likely than those with lower cholesterol levels to die suddenly. Under these circumstances, a comparison of surviving myocardial infarction patients against controls will underestimate the true association between total serum cholesterol elevation and risk of myocardial infarction.

Another potential type of selection bias can occur when a case-control study involves subjects who are hospitalized. Patients with two medical conditions are more likely to be hospitalized than those with a single disease. Thus, a hospital-based case-control study might find a link between two diseases or between an exposure and a disease when there was no association between them in the general population. This type of bias, often called Berkson's bias, was demonstrated in a study that showed that respiratory and bone diseases were associated in a sample of hospitalized patients but not in the general population. Thus, in a hospital-based study, an exposure such as cigarette smoking, which is correlated with respiratory disease, may also appear to occur together with bone disease because those diseases are related in hospitalized patients.

## Information Bias

*Information (or misclassification) bias can occur when there is random or systematic inaccuracy in measurement.* This can be visualized best in epidemiological studies that involve dichotomous exposure and disease variables, such as elevated total serum cholesterol and myocardial infarction. Subjects are classified according to whether or not they had high cholesterol and whether or not they had a myocardial infarction. The investigator either can be correct or incorrect, resulting in true-positive and true-negative as well as false-positive and false-negative classification of subjects with respect to either exposure or disease.

If the errors in classification of exposure or disease status are independent of the level of the other variable, then the misclassification is termed nondifferential. Nondifferential misclassification may occur in a case-control study if the subject's memory of exposure status is unrelated to whether or not the subject has the disease of interest. An example of nondifferential misclassification is sometimes referred to as unacceptability bias. Subjects may answer a question about the exposure with a socially acceptable but sometimes inaccurate response whether or not they have the disease of interest. Consider a case-control study of myocardial infarction in which the exposure of interest is prior intake of foods high in saturated fats. Regardless of disease status, respondents may underreport intake of foods with high fat content because they think low-fat diets are more acceptable to the investigator. In most instances when nondifferen-

tial misclassification occurs, it blurs differences between the study groups, making it more difficult for the investigator to detect an association between the exposure and the disease. This is often referred to as a bias toward the null hypothesis or toward no association.

Differential misclassification occurs when the misclassification of one variable depends upon the status of the other. In a case-control study, this type of misclassification could occur if the information on exposure status depended on whether or not the subject had the disease. If a case with a myocardial infarction is more likely to overestimate the level of dietary fat intake than a control subject, then a biased result might be found. In this instance, the bias would lead to an overestimate of the relationship between dietary fat intake and myocardial infarction.

The difference between nondifferential and differential misclassification can be demonstrated by examining the data in Figure 10–7. Consider a case-control study of the relationship between high-fat diets and myocardial infarction in which the true odds ratio (OR) is 2.3. With nondifferential misclassification, the subjects did not recall the amount of fatty foods eaten, but the errors in recall did not depend upon whether they had a myocardial infarction. In this situation, 20% of both cases and controls who ate high-fat diets underreported fat intake. The resulting OR of 2.0 was an underestimate of the true OR. On the other hand, if all the myocardial infarction patients correctly recalled their dietary fat exposure status but only 80% of the exposed controls correctly reported

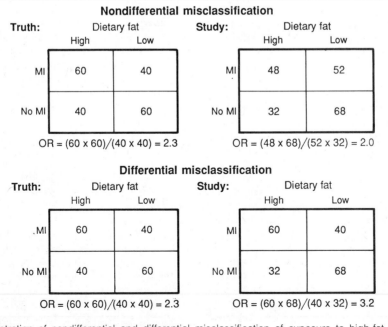

**Figure 10–7.** Illustration of nondifferential and differential misclassification of exposure to high-fat diets in a case-control study of myocardial infarction (MI). (OR = odds ratio.)

their exposure, then there would be differential misclassification. This type of misclassification can result in either an under- or overestimate of the true OR. In this example, the investigator overestimated the OR.

Two common types of differential information bias are often referred to as **recall bias** and **interviewer bias.** Recall bias results from differential ability of subjects to remember previous activities and exposures. Patients who have a serious disease may search their memory for an exposure in an attempt to explain or understand why they acquired the illness. Control subjects who do not have the disease may be less likely to remember an exposure because it has less meaning and is less important for them.

When interviewers are employed to determine exposures in case-control studies, results may be influenced by how they collect information. If interviewers know the research hypothesis, then they may influence the responses of the subjects. They may probe more deeply for responses from cases than from controls. If a dietary exposure is examined, the interviewers may ask certain subjects specific questions about particular food items. Interviewers may also give the subjects subtle clues by tone of voice or body language that suggest a preference for certain responses. Generally, it is desirable to blind the interviewers to the research hypothesis under investigation. In a case-control study, however, it may be difficult to blind the interviewers to the disease status of cases and controls. Nevertheless, if the interviewers are not aware of the exposure of primary interest, biased data collection still can be minimized.

## Confounding

*Confounding refers to the mixing of the effect of an extraneous variable with the effects of the exposure and disease of interest.* Confounding can be demonstrated by the following example. Suppose, for example, that a case-control study is undertaken of the association between high total serum cholesterol level and myocardial infarction. From the results of other studies, it is known that the risk of myocardial infarction is associated with obesity and that total cholesterol levels correlate with obesity (see Figure 10–8). In this case-control study, 36 of 60 (60%) of patients with myocardial infarction had high total cholesterol levels, and only 24 of 60 (40%) controls had elevated cholesterol levels. This suggests that elevated total cholesterol levels are associated with an increased risk of myocardial infarction.

When the observed association is examined separately in obese and nonobese persons, however, a different conclusion is reached. Among obese persons, 34 of 40 (85%) patients with myocardial infarction and 18 of 20 (90%) controls had elevated total cholesterol levels. Among nonobese persons, two of 20 (10%) patients with myocardial infarction and six of 40 (15%) controls had high total cholesterol levels.

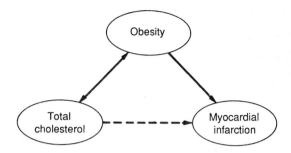

**Figure 10–8.** Schematic diagram of the relationship between total serum cholesterol level and risk of myocardial infarction, with confounding by obesity.

Elevated total cholesterol levels were more common in controls than in patients with myocardial infarction in both obese and nonobese individuals. It should be noted that in the hypothetical study, obesity was associated with myocardial infarction, since 52 of 60 (87%) obese subjects had elevated total cholesterol levels, and only eight of 60 (13%) nonobese persons had high cholesterol levels. The study results are shown diagrammatically in Figure 10–9.

For a variable to be considered a potential confounder, it must satisfy two conditions: (1) association with the disease of interest in the absence of exposure and (2) association with the exposure but not as a consequence of the exposure.

Since confounding can be evaluated in the analysis of results, it differs from selection bias and information bias. The presence of confounding is demonstrated by a change in the apparent strength of association between the exposure and the disease of interest when the effects of extraneous variables are taken into account. Confounding, which is not an all-or-none property of an extraneous variable, may occur to different degrees in different studies.

Generally, the list of potential confounders in a study is limited to established risk factors for the disease of interest. There are two accepted methods for dealing with potential confounders. The first is to consider them in the design of the study by matching on the potential confounder or restricting the sample to limited levels of the potential confounder. The other method is to evaluate confounding in the analysis by stratification, as demonstrated schematically in Figure 10–9, or by using multivariate analysis techniques such as multiple logistic regression.

The goal of any epidemiologic study is to provide a valid conclusion. In order to accomplish this objective, complete attention must be given to all aspects of the study, from inception through design and data collection to analysis and final reporting of results. Bias can be introduced at any of these stages, leading to erroneous results. It is useful to look for potential sources of bias and to consider their possible impact. Clinicians must judge whether results can be gener-

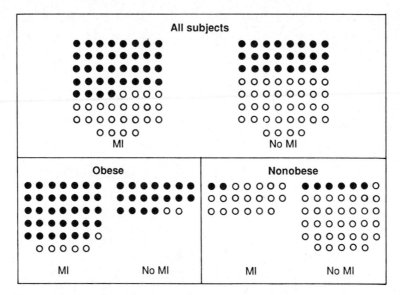

**Figure 10–9.** Illustration of the relationship between total serum cholesterol level and risk of myocardial infarction, with confounding by obesity. Shaded circles represent persons with elevated total serum cholesterol levels and unshaded circles represent persons with normal cholesterol levels.

alized to their particular practice. Understanding the potential problems with measurement and bias in medical research improves the physicians' ability to decide on appropriate preventive and therapeutic strategies.

## SUMMARY

In this chapter, the topics of variability and systematic errors in epidemiologic measurements were discussed, with illustrative examples primarily focused upon the relationship between total serum cholesterol and risk of myocardial infarction. A distinction was drawn between random variation, which is inversely related to precision in measurement, and nonrandom or systematic error, which is related to a distortion in measurement.

Variability can arise from the subjects under study, differences between individuals, the approach used to sample subjects, or the measurement process per se. Variability related to sampling is likely to diminish as the sample size increases. With extremely large sample sizes, a very small difference in outcome between study groups can be statistically significant. Whether the magnitude of this difference is sufficient to warrant a change in clinical practice is a separate, but equally important, question.

*Validity concerns the extent to which the findings of a study reflect truth.* **Internal validity** relates to the accuracy of study findings for the persons who were investigated. **External validity** concerns the extent to

which study findings accurately apply to persons who were not studied.

**Bias** is defined as lack of validity. Conventionally, bias is classified into three major types: **selection bias, information (misclassification) bias,** and **confounding.** Selection bias refers to the introduction of systematic errors into study results through the manner in which study subjects were selected. Information bias results in systematic errors in study findings that originate in the approach to collecting information. Two kinds of information bias have been described. **Nondifferential misclassification** occurs when errors in the information about one variable are unrelated to the status of another variable. **Differential misclassification,** on the other hand, occurs when errors in the information about one variable are affected by the status of another variable.

Confounding is concerned with the mixing of the primary effect of interest with the effects of one or more extraneous factors. In experimental studies, the problem of confounding is reduced by randomization, which tends to balance the study groups with respect to both known and unknown determinants of the outcome. In observational research, however, the study groups may differ appreciably in factors that are related to the risk of disease among unexposed persons and also associated with the exposure of interest. The influence of these potential confounders can be addressed in the study design (eg, through matching or restrictive inclusion criteria) or in the analysis (eg, through stratification or regression techniques). Only known confounders can be addressed in observational research.

No study is immune from the possibility of bias. The investigator must therefore consider potential sources of bias when sampling subjects, collecting information, analyzing results, and interpreting findings. With planning and forethought, it is possible to anticipate and avoid certain types of error and thus conduct a study that leads to a convincing and valid conclusion.

## STUDY QUESTIONS

**Directions:** For each question, select the single best answer.

**Questions 1–3:** A case-control study of aspirin use and myocardial infarction results in an odds ratio of 0.7 with an approximate 95% confidence interval of 0.3 to 1.3.

1. At the 5% level of statistical significance, the observed result is most appropriately interpreted as indicating a:
   A. Significant hazard
   B. Significant benefit
   C. Nonsignificant hazard
   D. Nonsignificant benefit

2. If the sample size was doubled and the same basic effect was observed, the approximate 95% confidence interval is most likely to be which of the following?
   A. 0.3 to 1.3
   B. 0.3 to 0.7
   C. 0.5 to 0.9
   D. 0.1 to 2.1
   E. 1.3 to 2.9

3. In a cohort study, the true risk ratio was 2.5, and the study had a bias away from the null hypothesis. The study risk ratio was most likely to be which of the following?
   A. 0.25
   B. 0.75
   C. 1.0
   D. 2.5
   E. 4.0

4. In a case-control study of maternal cigarette smoking as a hazard for low birth weight, it appeared that false-positive reports of cigarette smoking were more common among mothers of children of low birth weight than among mothers of children with normal birth weights. The reporting error most likely caused the odds ratio to:
   A. Increase
   B. Decrease
   C. Remain unchanged
   D. Change, but direction was uncertain

5. Among patients with oral cancer, alcohol drinkers have a worse prognosis than non-drinkers. When compared with a case-control study based upon incident cases only, a case-control study utilizing prevalent cases of oral cancer would likely have which of the following effects on the association between alcohol use and elevated risk of developing oral cancer?
   A. Increase
   B. Decrease
   C. Remain unchanged
   D. Change, but direction is uncertain

6. In a case-control study of the relationship between obesity and diabetes mellitus, controls are matched to cases on the basis of race and gender. This approach to subject selection is intended to decrease the chance of which of the following biases?
   A. Selection bias
   B. Ecologic fallacy
   C. Nondifferential misclassification
   D. Differential misclassification
   E. Confounding

**Questions 7–9:** In a case-control study of sunlight exposure and risk of cataracts, cases and controls were asked about participation in various outdoor activities and the use of eye protection. Errors in recall of exposure occurred with equal frequency among cases and controls.

7. Which one of the following biases occurred?
   A. Selection bias
   B. Ecologic fallacy
   C. Nondifferential misclassification
   D. Differential misclassification
   E. Confounding

8. The most likely effect of this bias on the risk estimation process was:
   A. Underestimation
   B. Overestimation
   C. No effect
   D. Cannot be determined

9. Which of the following approaches to adjustment of potential confounders is most likely to affect the external validity of a study?
   A. Randomization
   B. Restricted sampling
   C. Stratified analysis
   D. Regression analysis

10. In a cohort study of cigarette smoking as a hazard for bladder cancer, smokers with bladder cancer tended to die of other causes before the bladder cancer was diagnosed. This tendency was expected to have what effect on the association of interest?
    A. Underestimation
    B. Overestimation
    C. No effect
    D. Change, but direction was uncertain

## FURTHER READING

Rosenbaum PR: Discussing hidden bias in observational studies. Ann Intern Med 1991;115:90.

## REFERENCES

Devesa SS, Silverman DT: Cancer incidence and mortality trends in the United States, 1935–1974. J Natl Cancer Inst 1978;60:545.

Ellenberg JH, Nelson KB: Sample selection and the natural history of disease: Studies of febrile seizures. JAMA 1980;243:1337.

Report of the National Cholesterol Education Program Expert Panel on detection, evaluation and treatment of high blood cholesterol in adults. Arch Intern Med 1988; 148:36.

Horwitz RI, Feinstein AR: Methodologic standards and contradictory results in case-control research. Am J Med 1979;66:556.

Lipid Research Clinic Program: The Lipid Research Clinic's Coronary Primary Prevention Trial results. 1. Reduction in incidence of coronary heart disease. JAMA 1984;251:351.

National Heart, Lung and Blood Institute: *Recommendations for improving cholesterol measurements: A report from the laboratory standardization panel of the National Cholesterol Education Program.* US Department of Health and Human Services. NIH Publication No. 90–2964, 1990.

Roberts RS, Spitzer WO, Delmore T et al: Empirical demonstration of Berkson's bias. J Chron Dis 1978;31:119.

# Interpretation of Epidemiologic Literature

# 11

## PATIENT PROFILE

*A 40-year-old accountant was seen by her family physician for a routine checkup. The patient's mother had been diagnosed with breast cancer in the past year, and the patient wanted advice about what she could do to reduce her own risk of this disease. The patient had children aged 6 and 8 years. She was in good health, with regular menstrual cycles, and she had a recent normal Papanicolaou smear and mammogram.*

*In responding to the patient's questions about breast cancer, the physician confirmed that a positive family history does increase the risk of this disease. A number of other characteristics are associated with a reduced risk of breast cancer, such as early age at first full-term pregnancy and increasing number of pregnancies. Unfortunately, these factors are not easily susceptible to intervention, and the patient already had completed her childbearing. The physician was aware also of a controversy regarding the relationship between the intake of dietary fat and the occurrence of breast cancer. Before recommending that the patient reduce her fat intake, however, the physician wished to review the pertinent medical literature.*

## INTRODUCTION

The recommendations that physicians make to patients depend on the current state of knowledge available about diseases, the underlying pathophysiology, and the most effective treatment. The knowledge base of clinical medicine is continuously expanding, and physicians must therefore develop methods to seek out and apply new information. This process is complicated when inconclusive or conflicting results are found in the medical literature. The publication of articles, even in the most respected journals, does not guarantee that the investigators' conclusions are valid or, even if valid, relevant to the daily practice of a particular physician. The history of medicine includes countless examples of therapies that were once widely accepted but later were shown to be ineffec-

tive or even harmful to patients. Clinicians must develop skills that will allow them to update and reevaluate their knowledge in order to provide optimal patient care.

## SEARCHING THE LITERATURE

The first step in acquiring new medical knowledge is to locate the appropriate literature. This is an increasingly difficult task as the number of medical journals increases each year. It is not possible for any physician to read everything relevant to his or her practice as it is published. Fortunately, help of various kinds is available to assist with literature searching when necessary. A search of the existing literature can be performed manually, by reviewing keyword listings in the annual published indexes of the medical literature, such as *Index Medicus*. Examples of keywords that might be searched in the present context include "breast neoplasms," "dietary fats," and "food habits." In reviewing listings in *Index Medicus*, one is limited to information about the authors' names, the titles of the articles, and the journal, volume number and issue number, page numbers, and year of publication.

With the advent of computer technology, it has become possible to search the medical literature in an automated manner. For example, a search through a standard database, such as Medline, could be performed to assemble lists of articles that might be of interest. Again, the search process is based upon a few keywords chosen to recover articles on relevant subjects. Most computer databases include abstracts of articles from major journals, and some even include the entire text of articles from selected publications.

A computer search for the title words "breast cancer and dietary fat" retrieved a substantial number of journal articles over a recent 2-year period. These articles included case series, ecologic studies, descriptive studies, case-control studies, cohort studies, randomized controlled clinical trials, and reviews, including meta-analyses.

## CRITICAL REVIEW

Once the appropriate literature is identified, it is useful to apply a systematic approach to evaluating the articles. This process will encourage the reader to consider all aspects of a study before passing judgment on its validity and utility. The following sections provide one such approach to published studies. The steps in the review are presented in Figure 11–1 in the general sequence in which they should be considered. Each component of a review is dependent on the others to some extent, however, so that they are often considered collectively. The details of the review process are outlined in Table 11–1.

### Research Hypothesis

It is important to consider the research hypothesis that is addressed by the study. In practice, this may be a difficult task. Authors often do not state the hypotheses they wish to test. Sometimes the goal of the study is stated as a research question, but occasionally a reader is left to infer the purpose of the study from a set of complicated analyses.

Once the purpose of the study is discerned, the reader should attempt to determine if it addresses a question that has clinical importance. If it does not, the results may have little relevance to clinical practice. For the physician who needs information in or-

der to counsel a patient about the relationship of dietary fat and risk of breast cancer, it is necessary to identify articles that address that topic. A number of different kinds of hypotheses, however, may be relevant to the general topic. For example, a study of the

**Table 11–1.** Stepwise approach to critical appraisal of published medical research.

**Step 1. Consider the research hypothesis**
Is there a clear statement of the research hypothesis?
Does the study address a question that has clinical relevance?
**Step 2. Consider the study design**
Is the study design appropriate for the hypothesis?
Does the design represent an advance over prior approaches?
Does the study use an experimental or an observational design?
**Step 3. Consider the outcome variable**
Is the outcome being studied relevant to clinical practice?
What criteria are used to define the presence of disease?
Is the determination of the presence or absence of disease accurate?
**Step 4. Consider the predictor variable(s)**
How many exposures or risk factors are being studied?
How is the presence or absence of exposure determined? Is the assessment of exposure likely to be precise and accurate?
Is there an attempt to quantify the amount or duration of exposure?
Are biologic markers of exposure used in the study?
**Step 5. Consider the methods of analysis**
Are the statistical methods employed suitable for the types of variables (nominal versus ordinal versus continuous) in the study?
Have the levels of type I and type II errors been discussed appropriately?
Is the sample size adequate to answer the research question?
Have the assumptions underlying the statistical tests been met?
Has chance been evaluated as a potential explanation of the results?
**Step 6. Consider possible sources of bias (systematic errors)**
Is the method of selection of subjects likely to have biased the results?
Is the measurement of either the exposure or the disease likely to be biased?
Have the investigators considered whether confounders could account for the observed results?
In what direction would each potential bias influence the results?
**Step 7. Consider the interpretation of results**
How large is the observed effect?
Is there evidence of a dose-response relationship?
Are the findings consistent with laboratory models?
Are the effects biologically plausible?
If the findings are negative, was there sufficient statistical power to detect an effect?
**Step 8. Consider how the results of the study can be used in practice**
Are the findings consistent with other studies of the same questions?
Can the findings be generalized to other human populations?
Do the findings warrant a change in current clinical practice?

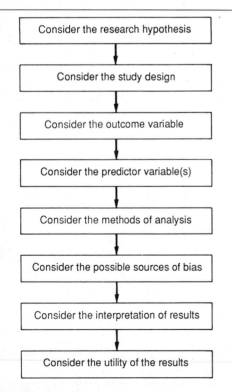

**Figure 11–1.** Steps in the evaluation of an epidemiologic study.

effects of varying dietary fat composition on the occurrence of mammary tumors in mice may be useful, because laboratory animal studies can be more tightly controlled than human studies. It may be useful to read a study on the effect of high-fat diet on circulating estrogen levels in women, since this may have relevance to the biologic plausibility of a potential relationship between dietary fat and breast cancer and may yield information about the mechanism of disease development and prevention.

The various types of **significance** that may be ascribed to a research finding should be distinguished (Table 11–2). It is common practice to refer to results as significant if a statistical test indicates that the findings are unlikely to be attributable to chance alone. The evaluation of statistical significance—and therefore the likelihood of committing a type I (false-positive) error—is useful in the interpretation of results.

Even if a finding is statistically significant, however, one cannot infer that it is biologically or clinically important. For instance, a small difference in risk of breast cancer with increasing levels of dietary fat could be judged to be statistically significant if it were based upon a large number of observations. Nevertheless, this elevation in risk may be so small that an individual woman's risk of breast cancer would not be appreciably altered by changing her diet. As a result, a clinical recommendation to reduce dietary fat might not be supportable on the basis of the evidence. The biologic significance of a finding addresses yet another issue: Do the epidemiologic observations help to clarify the causal mechanism? This type of insight is most likely to be gained if the epidemiologic study involves biologic markers of exposure, susceptibility, and outcome.

## Study Design

If the study question is of interest, the reader should then determine what type of study design was employed. As was noted in Chapters 7–9, certain designs may be more or less useful for answering specific kinds of questions. Another factor that may have determined the type of study design used by the investigator is the current state of knowledge. Early studies of a particular hypothesis may have a simple design, such as a descriptive study. As the hypothesis is refined, more definitive study designs can be utilized.

The appropriateness of the study design to the research question should be assessed. The incidence rate of the disease in question may be a determining factor. For example, although breast cancer is the most common form of cancer among women in the United States, this disease is diagnosed among only a small proportion of women during a short period of time. Accordingly, an appropriate choice of design for this disease would be a case-control study, since the sampling scheme for this type of study is efficient for including newly diagnosed women. In fact, studies of dietary fat intake and breast cancer have utilized several different designs, including descriptive, case-control, and cohort studies. The descriptive studies are most useful for hypothesis generation. The case-control and cohort designs provide more compelling evidence for testing specific hypotheses. To date, all of the studies of dietary fat and risk of breast cancer have employed observational designs. An experimental study in which women are assigned randomly to groups receiving different levels of dietary fat and followed for the occurrence of breast cancer has not yet been performed. This type of study would represent an important future step in examining a possible causal relationship between dietary fat intake and breast cancer.

## Outcome Variable

The outcome of interest in the Patient Profile is breast cancer. In investigations of the relationship between dietary fat intake and risk of breast cancer, it is important to specify how the presence or absence of breast cancer was determined. There are several possibilities.

**(1)** Death certificates limit information to deceased subjects. In addition, a variety of studies have shown that information on death certificates may be incomplete or inaccurate.

**(2)** Self-reports require that subjects be alive or have relatives who can provide information on breast cancer. If the subjects are not medically sophisticated, they may mistake benign forms of breast disease for breast cancer.

**(3)** Medical records may provide more accurate information. However, it is possible that diagnostic criteria differ from physician to physician, that they may change over time, or that there may be differences in different geographic regions in international studies.

**(4)** Histopathologic diagnoses provide the most definitive information, but adequate tissue must be available for pathologic examination.

**Table 11–2.** Types of significance in clinical research.

| Type | Meaning | Assessment |
|------|---------|------------|
| Statistical | Exclusion of chance as an explanation for findings | Statistical test |
| Clinical | Importance of findings for changing current clinical practice | Magnitude of clinical response to an intervention |
| Biologic | Findings help to clarify mechanism of action | Compare findings to information from in vitro and in vivo laboratory experimentation |

It is desirable to have the most definitive information possible on the presence of disease. This will tend to minimize the likelihood of misclassification of subjects. For breast cancer, it is possible that a small proportion of apparently healthy women may actually have occult (undiscovered) breast cancer. This could be evaluated by performing a screening test, such as mammography, on all apparently unaffected subjects. Since so few asymptomatic cancers are likely to be detected, however, study findings probably would not be affected greatly by limiting detection to routine histopathologic diagnosis.

It is also important to judge how precisely the investigator defines the outcome. In general, it is useful to specify a single disease entity when searching for causes. For example, a study of dietary fat and the risk of all cancers combined may produce misleading results, since different cancers have different causes, some of which may include dietary fat. Restricting the study to breast cancer improves the likelihood of obtaining a definitive result.

## Predictor Variables

The predictor variable is the risk factor or exposure that is under investigation. Studies may involve a single risk factor of interest or several different predictor variables. If a number of exposure variables are included, they may or may not be closely linked.

In a study of the cause of breast cancer, an investigator might choose to examine a variety of exposure variables, including reproductive factors such as age at first full-term pregnancy, hormone levels, exposure to radiation, and dietary fat intake. While this sort of study may provide a more comprehensive picture of the causes of breast cancer, it may limit the ability to collect detailed information on each exposure of interest. Even if a study is focused on the question of dietary fat and the risk of breast cancer, it is necessary to collect some basic information on other possible determinants of breast cancer that could act as confounders.

The reader must determine whether the methods used to characterize the presence or absence of exposure are reliable and accurate. Possible ascertainment methods include subject or surrogate respondent reports, direct observation, or measurement of a biologic marker. The reader should ask whether there are better ways to define the exposure levels of subjects.

The assessment of a dietary exposure can be especially difficult. One method would be to ask subjects about their past dietary habits. This requires that the subjects remember both the kinds and the amounts of foods that they ate. A variety of studies have indicated that such recall is imperfect but that it may be sufficient to allow a determination of whether a subject consumed a relatively high, moderate, or low amount of dietary fat. Generally, it is desirable to have several levels of exposure defined, so that a dose-response relationship can be evaluated.

Another approach to determining dietary fat intake would be to have subjects record what they currently eat. This can be done by keeping a diary or by checking off the types of foods eaten on a food frequency list. Problems with this approach are that subjects may forget to record what they eat or incorrectly estimate the size of portions. Plastic models of different portion sizes have been used to provide visual cues. It is important to remember that a subject's current diet may not accurately reflect past diet. In a case-control design based only upon current diet information, it would be crucial to know if subjects with breast cancer perhaps changed their diets as a consequence of the disease, the side effects of treatment, or in hope of influencing prognosis.

Another approach to collecting information on diet would be to measure what subjects eat. This could be useful for a prospective cohort study in which subjects are followed to determine if they do or do not develop breast cancer. This approach to measuring dietary intake would be extremely difficult in practice, however, as it would require a tightly controlled environment in which the investigator could observe the foods eaten by subjects.

Epidemiologists occasionally take advantage of a situation in which people maintain certain dietary habits for religious or other reasons. Thus, an epidemiologist may identify a group of people (eg, vegetarians) who, because of their beliefs, consume very little fat. The frequency of occurrence of breast cancer in this group then could be compared with the experience of another group in which large amounts of fat are consumed. The problem of determining the precise intake of fat for subjects in both groups still remains, however. Furthermore, it is likely that the groups will differ in life-style factors other than intake of dietary fat.

The use of biologic markers of exposure has become more common in clinical research. Biologic markers are important because they can provide quantitative documentation of exposure in certain circumstances. No biologic markers of fat intake are currently available, but in order to assess long-term dietary fat intake, one might measure fatty acid content in biopsies of adipose tissue. Obviously, the utility of such a measure depends upon the extent to which it accurately reflects consumption patterns. The willingness of study participants to undergo a tissue biopsy must also be considered.

## Methods of Analysis

The emphasis that is placed on a particular research finding often depends on the ability of the investigator to exclude chance as an explanation for the observed results. This is accomplished by the use of statistical tests. It is important for the reader to have a basic understanding of which statistical tests are appropriate for which types of analysis. The type of statistical test that should be used is determined by the goal of the analysis (eg, comparing groups, exploring an association, or predicting) and the types of variables used in the analysis (eg, categorical, ordinal, or continuous).

By convention, the 5% level of statistical significance is used as a standard in many biomedical studies. That is, the investigator is willing to accept a one in 20 risk that the observed effect is a result of chance variation alone. Care must be taken to avoid oversimplistic interpretations of $P$-values, however. One common mistake is to assume that a statistically significant result is biologically or clinically important. As discussed above, the clinical and biologic importance of results is not assessed by hypothesis tests.

A second common mistake is to dismiss a finding because it has not reached the predetermined level for statistical significance. A $P$-value of 0.08, for example, though not statistically significant by ordinary criteria, still represents a finding that is relatively unlikely to be attributable to chance. The heavy reliance upon $P$-values is particularly dangerous when the sample size is small and the statistical power therefore is low as well. In that situation, even moderate differences between groups may fail to reach a standard level of statistical significance, and the ability to reach a definitive conclusion is limited.

## Possible Sources of Bias

A result must be examined also to determine whether it could be due to systematic errors related to the sampling strategy or data collection procedures. A statistical test cannot address the question whether biases of one sort or another are responsible for the observed results. As discussed in Chapter 10, the consideration of potential bias is subjective. Bias can occur in any study, although certain designs are more susceptible to specific types of bias. Regardless of the study design, the potential for three distinct types of bias should be considered (Table 11–3).

The first concern is whether the selection of subjects is likely to have distorted the results (**selection bias**). Few studies (if any) can examine an entire population. This means that the investigator must draw a sample in order to make inferences about the population. The reader must determine if the samples are likely to be representative of the population to which extrapolations are made.

The methods section of any published medical research paper should include details of how subjects were selected for the study. In a case-control study, selection bias could arise from the approach used to select cases, controls, or both. In the context of a case-control study of dietary fat and breast cancer, selection bias might occur if prevalent (surviving) cases are used rather than newly diagnosed (incident) cases. This distortion would occur if prediagnostic nutritional status were related to disease prognosis. For example, if women who consumed high-fat diets before developing breast cancer survived longer than low-fat consumers, prevalent cases would overrepresent high-fat consumption, and the observed risk ratio may be biased toward larger values. The bias is presented schematically in Figure 11–2.

In a case-control study, the sampling of controls can be as great a source of selection bias as the sampling of cases. Consider a hospital-based sample of controls with diagnoses other than breast cancer. If the diseases of the controls are caused by dietary factors (eg, atherosclerotic heart disease)—or, conversely, if the diseases influence dietary intake (eg, gastrointestinal disease)—a biased case-control comparison may result. Alternatively, selection of controls from the general population can lead to bias. For example, a telephone sampling technique might pref-

**Table 11–3.** Types of bias in clinical research.

| Bias | Source of Error |
|---|---|
| Selection bias | Sample distorted by selection process |
| Information bias | Misclassification of the variables |
| Confounding | An extraneous variable that accounts for the observed result rather than the risk factor of interest |

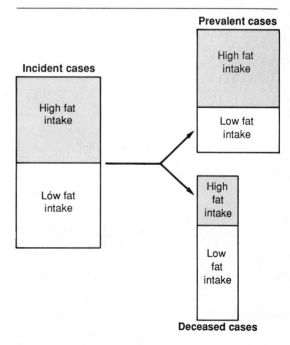

**Figure 11–2.** Schematic diagram of bias introduced by study of prevalent cases when the risk factor (high fat intake) is related to prognosis. Shaded areas represent cases with high fat intake and unshaded areas represent cases with low fat intake. Note that the deceased cases included a relatively large proportion of persons taking diets low in fat, resulting in overrepresentation of high-fat consumers among the prevalent cases.

erentially include higher-income women, ie, those who do not work outside the home. Since the diets of these women may differ from those of other women, a biased case-control comparison may occur.

Cohort studies of the association between dietary factors and breast cancer also are subject to potential selection bias. The major source of selection bias in such studies is loss to follow-up during the study. If women who eat a high-fat diet and develop breast cancer tend to discontinue participation in the study for some reason prior to the diagnosis of cancer, the investigator will underestimate the risk for breast cancer associated with a high-fat intake. To date, cohort studies of this question have yielded conflicting results. An important consideration in such a situation is the extent to which bias due to loss to follow-up could explain the discrepancy.

Another source of bias can arise from systematic errors in measuring either the independent variable (exposure) or the dependent variable (disease). This type of bias is often referred to as **information bias** or **misclassification bias.** For example, in a case-control study, the validity of information on exposure may be questioned because the data are gathered retrospectively. Since the cases are aware of their disease and have undergone treatment for it, their reporting of past exposures may differ systematically from reporting of controls. This is referred to as **recall bias.** Studies of dietary risk factors may be susceptible to recall bias. For example, if breast cancer patients are wondering about the cause of their cancer, they may tend to overestimate past exposure to dietary fat, especially when the potential relationship has been widely publicized. Controls may be less concerned about past diet or may be worried about other problems such as obesity, which would tend to make them underreport exposure to dietary fat.

If recall bias occurred in a study, the investigator might overestimate the risk of dietary fat intake in relation to the occurrence of breast cancer. In fact, a number of studies have demonstrated problems of imperfect recall of dietary history. However, only a few studies have examined differential (biased) recall in cases versus control subjects by comparing prospectively collected dietary data with subsequent data collected retrospectively from the same subjects. In general, these investigations have not demonstrated differential recall of food intake in breast cancer cases compared with controls. This would suggest that recall bias is an unlikely explanation for inconsistent results reported from case-control studies of the association of dietary fat intake and breast cancer.

It should be remembered, however, that even if cases and controls do not differ in their ability to recall dietary exposure, misclassification bias could still occur. Errors in reporting that are comparable between cases and controls give rise to nondifferential misclassification. If nondifferential misclassification does occur, it may reduce the estimated risk ratio. In

other words, such misclassification tends to blur differences between cases and controls.

The final consideration of bias is to determine whether **confounding** could account for the observed result. A confounder is an extraneous correlate of disease that, because of its association with the risk factor of interest, accounts for some or all of the observed association between the risk factor and the disease. In studies of dietary fat intake and breast cancer, it would be important to determine if the investigator accounted for the effects of known risk factors for breast cancer. These factors would include age, race, reproductive characteristics (eg, age at first full-term pregnancy, number of pregnancies, duration of lactation), obesity among postmenopausal women, alcohol intake, and exposure to radiation. A schematic diagram of confounding of the relationship between dietary fat intake and breast cancer by number of pregnancies is presented in Figure 11–3. If women who eat a high-fat diet have fewer pregnancies than those who eat a low-fat diet, an apparent association between dietary fat and breast cancer could be attributable to the effects of reproductive history rather than to diet per se.

Confounding can be controlled in an observational study either in the design (by restricting subject inclusion to persons with a narrow range of the confounder values, or by matching study groups on confounders) or in the analysis (through stratification by confounders, or by regression techniques). All of these adjustment methods, however, are contingent upon knowing which variables are confounders. Since the known risk factors for breast cancer do not account for all occurrences of the disease, other unknown risk factors must exist. Any observed association between dietary fat and breast cancer could be explained, at least in part, in that way.

When the reader detects the potential for bias, it is important to try to estimate both the magnitude and the direction of the effect the bias could have on the results. In this way, the reader can determine if the bias is likely to have inflated the results or actually may have diminished the effect. For example, if it is

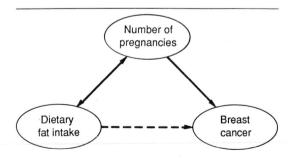

**Figure 11–3.** Schematic diagram of confounding of the dietary fat-breast cancer relationship by number of pregnancies.

suspected that women with breast cancer in a case-control study are more likely to remember and report fat intake than controls, the risk ratio could be overestimated. In contrast, if it seems likely that breast cancer patients underreport their dietary fat intake in comparison with controls, the observed results may underestimate the true impact of dietary fat intake on the occurrence of breast cancer. In discussing the results, an investigator may attempt to convince the reader that the magnitude of bias would not be sufficient to skew the results or that the true relationship is as strong as or stronger than that observed.

## Interpretation of Results

If the investigator reports a statistically significant result that cannot be explained by bias, the reader must then decide whether the result is clinically important. Consider, for example, a study concluding that a 50% decrease in dietary fat intake is associated with a 5% decrease in risk of breast cancer. Even if this result is statistically significant, the magnitude of risk reduction is so slight in exchange for the major change in diet that would be called for that the finding is unlikely to lead to a useful clinical intervention—although it may still have biologic significance if it provides insight into the mechanism of carcinogenesis.

Conversely, when results are not statistically significant, one need not conclude that the findings are not useful. Particularly when there is a small sample size or when the relationship between the exposure and the disease is weak, the possibility of a false-negative conclusion must be considered. The statistical power of the study to detect the observed effect may be too low to allow a definitive conclusion from the study.

## Practical Utility of Results

When reviewing a published study, the reader must determine the practical utility of the results. The usefulness of a study finding depends on a variety of factors, including the purpose of the study, limitations of the study population, the clinical and biologic importance of the results, and consistency with findings from other published studies. There are a variety of different purposes of clinical and epidemiologic research. The clinical utility of a particular research finding must be viewed in the context of the type of question posed. As indicated in Table 11–4, a particular study may lead to findings relevant to disease causation, early detection of disease, predicting prognosis, or improved treatment. Studies of the relationship between dietary fat and breast cancer relate to disease causation. Unfortunately, there is no standard by which to judge whether an association between risk factor and a disease is clinically important. Clearly, the stronger the association (ie, the farther the risk ratio is from the null value), the greater the potential impact of eliminating the exposure. In as-

**Table 11–4.** Clinical applications of various types of studies.

| Type of Study | Application to Clinical Practice |
|---|---|
| Etiologic | Can risk be reduced among susceptible persons? |
| Diagnostic | Can accuracy and timeliness of diagnosis be improved? |
| Prognostic | Can prognosis be determined more definitively? |
| Therapeutic | Can treatment be improved? |

sessing clinical utility, one must also consider how difficult it is to change the risk factor (ie, reduce dietary fat intake) as well as the amount of morbidity and mortality associated with the disease.

The ability to generalize the findings beyond the study population should be considered. For this purpose, the definition and limitations of the study sample must be understood. For example, some studies of risk factors for breast cancer have focused on postmenopausal women. This may limit the applicability of such studies to the premenopausal patient in the Patient Profile. Investigators are often forced to restrict the sample by age, race, or other factors. The reader must decide what effect these restrictions have on the applicability of results.

In determining whether the findings of a particular study can be generalized to other populations, it is useful to assess whether similar results have been obtained in other studies. It often happens that the first evaluation of a risk factor, diagnostic test, or therapeutic regimen is favorable, whereas subsequent reports demonstrate more limited utility. One reason for this pattern is that initial assessments often involve selected populations that offer a best-case scenario. Subsequent attempts to broaden the applicability may prove less successful.

## ESTABLISHING A CAUSAL RELATIONSHIP

Ultimately, the reader may question whether a causal relationship between a risk factor and a disease has been supported by the results of a study. In Table 11–5, selected criteria are presented that can be used to evaluate suspected causal relationships. The consideration of causality is based upon the findings of a

**Table 11–5.** Selected criteria for evaluating a suspected causal relationship.

Strength
Presence of a dose-response relationship
Correct temporal sequence
Consistency of results across studies
Biologic plausibility

particular study in the context of what is already known about the disease process.

The **strength of the observed association** is a primary criterion for evaluating whether a risk factor causes a disease. The strength of the association is indicated by the distance of the risk ratio or odds ratio from the null value. When the association is very strong, it is less likely that it can be explained by chance or bias. Weak associations also may be causal, indicating only a lower risk of disease development. With a weak association, however, it is more difficult to exclude other factors and biases that may account for the relationship.

It is useful to examine whether there is a **dose-response relationship** between the proposed risk factor and the disease. If one is present, increased levels of the risk factor will be associated with a greater risk of disease development (or protection for a beneficial factor). For example, as the level of dietary fat intake increases, the risk of breast cancer would be expected to increase if a causal relationship exists (Figure 11–4). The absence of a progressive, graded dose-response relationship does not preclude a causal relationship, however. For example, there may be a threshold above which the level of the risk factor confers increased risk. In this case, risk of disease will not be affected by changes in exposure below a certain level, but risk does vary with exposure at higher levels.

With any association, it is helpful to compare the findings with the results of other studies. If other investigators studying different populations in differing settings find similar results, a causal explanation is supported. However, the reader must be careful when judging consistency of results, because it is possible that the same flaw could lead to incorrect conclusions in several different studies.

The proposed causal relationship should be consistent with what is currently known about biology and the disease process. This is often referred to as **biologic plausibility.** If the proposed cause-and-effect relationship is not in accordance with current knowledge, causality may be questioned. The assessment of biologic plausibility often requires review of research on other human populations as well as laboratory animal models.

The temporal relationship between a suspected cause and an effect is important. That is, *a cause must always precede an effect in time.* This seems intuitive, but, in reality, factors that are suspected to be causes sometimes turn out to be effects of the disease. For example, a person with an early undiagnosed cancer may make a change in food choices because of unrecognized systemic effects of the cancer. As a consequence, a dietary change may appear to be the cause of the later diagnosed cancer rather than an effect of the cancer. Case-control studies of chronic diseases with long latent periods are especially susceptible to this problem. For a factor to be considered the cause of a disease, it is theoretically important that removal or modification of that factor will prevent the disease from occurring or ameliorate the disease once it has occurred. This criterion has been met for the example cited in Chapter 9, since the incidence of Reye's syndrome has declined with decreased use of aspirin to treat symptoms associated with viral illnesses in children. In practice, however, this criterion may not always be satisfied. There are some instances where a causal factor may set off a protracted chain of events. Once established, this sequence may no longer depend on the presence of the causal agent for progression. For example, many cancers are thought to develop in response to an initiating event, followed by promotional effects that occur for many years. If the risk factor of interest contributes to initiation only, removal of the exposure during the promotional phase will not affect the subsequent risk of cancer development. Thus, eliminating an initiating risk factor for cancer may not affect the incidence of this disease for many years into the future.

## DIETARY FAT AND BREAST CANCER

As mentioned previously, the relationship between dietary fat intake and the risk of breast cancer was investigated in a variety of epidemiologic studies. These studies included case series, ecologic analyses, case-control studies, and cohort studies. To date, no randomized controlled clinical trial of a low-fat diet to prevent breast cancer has been performed.

Ecologic or correlation studies showed a consistently strong relationship between dietary habits as estimated by per capita dietary fat and breast cancer

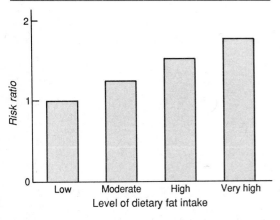

**Figure 11–4.** Hypothetical dose-response relationship between level of dietary fat intake and risk ratio of breast cancer. The reference category of exposure is low dietary fat intake.

occurrence in different countries. Plots of these data yielded a linear relationship, with increasing fat consumption associated with higher breast cancer occurrence. The problem with such studies is that they do not demonstrate that increased dietary fat in *individuals* is associated with breast cancer occurrence in the same *individuals* (ie, the **ecologic fallacy**).

Case-control studies yielded conflicting results on the question of diet and breast cancer. The reasons for these conflicting results are not clear. One criticism is that dietary data collected retrospectively are inaccurate (ie, misclassified exposure). Another potential explanation is that the influence of dietary fat could have been exerted many years prior to breast cancer diagnosis. Most case-control studies have included diet information from the recent past but not from the remote past. Some reviewers concluded that none of the studies individually were of large enough sample size to provide adequate statistical power. In other words, a true relationship between dietary fat intake and breast cancer risk might be missed because of inadequate discriminatory ability (ie, a type II error).

Some of these problems can be avoided with the cohort study design. Prospective cohort studies eliminate the potential for distortion of results from differential recall of dietary history. This type of investigation was used to investigate the question of fat in the diet and the risk of breast cancer. Again, the published results of cohort studies of this question yielded conflicting results. Some studies produced evidence of a relatively weak association, with risk ratios of approximately 1.4. However, other cohort studies actually indicated that increased dietary fat intake may protect against the development of breast cancer.

In general, the dose-response relationship suggested by the ecologic studies was not been borne out in the case-control and cohort studies. Some reviewers argued that the reason for this disagreement is that the range of dietary fat intake in the analytic studies is smaller than in the international ecologic studies—and, consequently, that there was too little variation in fat intake to demonstrate a dose-response relationship. Others argued that factors other than diet (ie, confounders) that could not be controlled easily in ecologic studies were the real explanation for the association between fat intake and breast cancer observed in correlation analyses.

In situations where the sample size is not adequate in individual studies to reach a firm conclusion, investigators sometimes combine the results of several studies. This pooling of data from several studies is referred to as **meta-analysis.** Meta-analysis can be useful for achieving greater statistical power, but it cannot overcome the limitations and potential biases of individual studies. The investigator performing a meta-analysis must also be careful that selection of some studies and exclusion of others does not lead to

a distorted conclusion. One meta-analysis of studies of diet and breast cancer combined the results from 12 case-control studies. No relationship between dietary fat intake and risk of breast cancer in premenopausal women was found, but an association between fat intake and breast cancer in postmenopausal women was detected, with a risk ratio of 1.5.

In the Patient Profile, the physician wanted to determine whether dietary fat intake is causally related to the development of breast cancer. The findings of studies were inconsistent, and the strength of association was modest at best, without clear evidence of a dose-response relationship. The temporal sequence of dietary fat intake and breast cancer appeared to be reasonable.

Was there biologic plausibility to the relationship? What pathophysiologic mechanism might be involved? Were there animal models that showed the relationship between fat in the diet and breast cancer? In fact, there were animal studies in which fat intake was associated with the development of mammary cancers in mice bearing the mammary tumor virus. Similar findings were reported in other animal models. The pathophysiology involved in this process was less clear, but potential mechanisms were discussed. There was speculation that mammary neoplasms were controlled by endocrine balance, which in turn was affected by dietary factors, including fat intake. For example, women taking high-fat diets were shown to have more circulating estrogen than women on low-fat diets. In postmenopausal women, adipose tissue was demonstrated to be a contributor to the production of estrogen. Dietary fat intake may also have modified DNA synthesis and cell duplication. If this was true for breast tissue, this could be relevant to breast carcinogenesis. Therefore, it did appear that there were some theoretical reasons to believe that a causal relationship existed between dietary fat intake and breast cancer.

The physician in the Patient Profile ultimately was left without a firm answer to the question about the relationship between dietary fat and breast cancer. Even if there was a small increase in risk with high-fat diets for postmenopausal women, the patient was premenopausal, so it was not clear that the results could be applied to this patient. On the other hand, it was only a matter of time before she would go through menopause. Dietary habits presumably would be continued and could be protective in later life. The physician also may have felt that a low-fat diet would be justifiable for other reasons, including reduction of risk for cardiovascular disease. In addition, there were other cancers, such as colon cancer, for which the protective effect of a low-fat diet was demonstrated more clearly.

This type of uncertainty is common in clinical medicine. Physicians often must weigh potential risks and benefits of an intervention and make decisions without complete information. The goal of medical research is to continue to provide better answers to important clinical questions. Perhaps the only way to resolve the issue of the relationship of dietary fat and breast cancer is to embark on a large randomized controlled trial to compare breast cancer occurrence in women randomized to a low-fat diet compared to those on a high-fat diet. Clearly, this type of study would provide the most definitive evidence about a causal relationship between dietary fat and risk of breast cancer. Such a study would require a large number of subjects and a long follow-up period. It could be argued that the resources required for this study would be better spent on studies of other questions where the evidence of a beneficial effect is stronger.

Much of the satisfaction derived from patient care relates to the ability to incorporate new knowledge into the practice of medicine. In order to update one's knowledge, it is imperative to develop the skills required for critical review of the medical literature. This is a difficult task, but the reward is enormous when it results in improved patient care.

## SUMMARY

In this chapter, a structured approach to reviewing published epidemiologic studies was presented. The ultimate goal of this approach is to help integrate epidemiologic information into clinical practice. As a focus for discussion, the literature on dietary fat intake and risk of breast cancer was used to illustrate the evaluation process.

The initial step in reviewing the medical literature is to conduct a thorough search for relevant recent publications. Screening for appropriate articles can be accomplished through a manual or a computer-assisted system. In either case, a correct choice of keywords calculated to retrieve pertinent articles is essential. Computer searches can save time and consequently are extremely popular.

The actual review of a publication begins with the stated purpose of the investigation. For the medical practitioner, a primary consideration is whether a particular study addresses a clinically important question. Are the results likely to influence the delivery of patient care? In the present context, clinical importance might be assessed in terms of whether the findings support a recommendation to lower dietary fat intake in order to reduce the risk of breast cancer.

The design of an investigation determines the types of inferences that can be drawn from it. The most compelling evidence for cause-and-effect relationships is derived from randomized controlled clinical trials. Among observational investigations, prospective cohort studies generally are least susceptible to bias, followed by retrospective cohort and case-control studies. Descriptive studies are useful for generating research questions but not for testing hypotheses.

The measurement of outcome (ie, development of disease) as well as the documentation of exposure to risk factors can be complicated in observational research. Emphasis must be placed on obtaining the most accurate information possible, recognizing that the ideal often cannot be achieved. Whenever possible, assessment should be performed in a blinded manner and should be based upon objective, standard criteria.

A distinction must be made between the concept of statistical significance, which can be evaluated by a hypothesis test, and clinical or biologic significance. $P$-values should not be used to indicate the importance of a finding but rather the likelihood that sampling variability could explain the results. Clinical importance relates to whether a difference in outcomes observed between study groups is large enough to warrant a change in clinical practice. Biologic significance refers to the extent to which findings help to elucidate the underlying biologic processes.

Systematic errors may arise in observational research from the approach to sample selection, information collection, or confounding. It is usually impossible to determine whether a particular bias actually occurred. Attention, therefore, is focused on strategies to minimize the likelihood that systematic errors will affect the study conclusions. When bias is suspected in an investigation, the exact level of distortion generally is unknown. The direction of the systematic error (ie, a tendency to either overestimate or underestimate the strength of association) may be clear, however. The assessment of whether an observed association is likely to be one of cause and effect is based upon specific criteria, including strength of association, presence of a dose-response relationship, appropriateness of the temporal sequence of exposure and outcome, consistency of results across studies, and biologic plausibility.

When applied to the literature on dietary fat and breast cancer, this process of reasoning leads to an inconclusive assessment. The most consistent supporting evidence comes from the least compelling types of study. In those situations where an association was observed, the magnitude generally was weak. Results were inconsistent across studies, perhaps due in part to limitations of the study design and in part to the weakness of the relationship, even if it does exist. The ultimate test of this hypothesis—a randomized controlled clinical trial—has not yet been performed.

As with many issues in medicine, the dietary fat-breast cancer hypothesis remains unresolved. Since little harm probably results from restriction of dietary fat intake and because other benefits may accrue (ie, a reduction in risk of cardiovascular disease), it may be reasonable for the clinician in the Patient Profile to recommend this change in dietary habits to the patient. Until more definitive information is available, however, the patient should be counseled that the effect of restricting dietary fat intake on the risk of breast cancer is uncertain.

## STUDY QUESTIONS

**Directions:** For each question, select the single best answer:

**Questions 1–2:** An investigator finds a positive correlation between per capita alcohol consumption and mortality rates for breast cancer across 20 different countries.

1. This type of study is most useful for:
   A. Hypothesis generation
   B. Hypothesis testing
   C. Assessing confounding
   D. Determining clinical importance
   E. Evaluating causality

2. If the individual women who develop breast cancer are not heavy drinkers, then the apparent positive correlation between national per capita alcohol consumption and breast cancer mortality most likely reflects:
   A. Recall bias
   B. Selection bias
   C. Ecologic fallacy
   D. Lack of complete disease registration
   E. Loss to follow-up

**Questions 3–4:** In order to investigate this relationship further, a study is conducted in which 200 women with breast cancer and 200 women without breast cancer are compared with respect to earlier drinking habits.

3. The design of this study is best described as:
   A. Ecologic
   B. Case-control
   C. Prospective cohort
   D. Retrospective cohort
   E. Randomized controlled clinical trial

4. If women with breast cancer are more likely than women without breast cancer to overestimate prior alcohol consumption, the apparent association between drinking and risk of breast cancer will be:
   A. Decreased
   B. Unchanged
   C. Altered, but the direction cannot be predicted
   D. Increased

**Questions 5–9:** Next, a study is conducted in which 10,000 women without breast cancer are enrolled, questioned about alcohol consumption, and then followed for future development of breast cancer.

5. The design of this study is best described as:
   A. Ecologic
   B. Case-control
   C. Prospective cohort
   D. Retrospective cohort
   E. Randomized controlled clinical trial

6. If heavy alcohol drinkers who develop cancer are selectively lost from this study prior to the diagnosis of breast cancer, the apparent association between alcohol drinking and risk of breast cancer will be:
   A. Decreased
   B. Unchanged
   C. Altered, but the direction cannot be predicted
   D. Increased

7. In this study, white females are more likely to drink than black females. White females also experience a higher risk of breast cancer. Failure to account for the effect of race could result in which of the following types of bias?
   A. Recall bias
   B. Selection bias
   C. Differential misclassification
   D. Nondifferential misclassification
   E. Confounding

8. If the risk ratio for breast cancer increases with reported level of alcohol consumption, it can be inferred that there is:
   A. A biologically plausible relationship
   B. A statistically significant result
   C. A clinically important finding
   D. A dose-response relationship
   E. A consistent relationship across studies

9. If the estimated risk ratio of heavy to light drinking is 1.5, with a 95% confidence interval of (1.1, 2.2), it can be inferred that there is:
   A. A biologically plausible relationship
   B. A statistically significant result
   C. A clinically important finding
   D. A dose-response relationship
   E. A consistent relationship across studies

10. The results of several analytic epidemiologic studies are combined into a summary comparison of the association between alcohol consumption and the risk of breast cancer. This summary is best described as:
    A. A cost-benefit analysis
    B. A decision analysis
    C. A correlation analysis
    D. A matched analysis
    E. A meta-analysis

## FURTHER READING

Willett W: The search for the causes of breast and colon cancer. Nature 1989;338:389.

## REFERENCES

Dawson-Saunders B, Trapp RG: Reading the medical literature. In: *Basic and Clinical Biostatistics.* Appleton & Lange, 1990.

Gehlbach SH: *Interpreting the Medical Literature,* 2nd ed. MacMillan, 1988.

Riegelman RK, Hirsch RP: Studying a study. In: *Studying a Study and Testing a Test,* 2nd ed. Little, Brown, 1989.

Sackett DL, Haynes RB, Tugwell P: How to read a clinical journal. In: *Clinical Epidemiology.* Little, Brown, 1985.

# Glossary

**Accuracy:** the extent to which a measurement or study result correctly represents the characteristic or relationship that is being assessed.

**Adjustment:** a procedure for overall comparison of two or more populations in which background differences in the distribution of covariables are removed. (See also **Standardization**.)

**Age adjustment:** a procedure used to calculate summary rates for different populations in which underlying differences in the age distributions are removed. (See also **Age standardization**.)

**Age-specific rate:** a rate (usually incidence or mortality) for a particular age group.

**Age standardization (direct):** a procedure for obtaining a weighted average of age-specific rates in which the weights are selected on the basis of a standard age distribution (eg, the population of the United States in 1940).

**Alpha error:** see **Type I error.**

**Analytic epidemiology:** activities related to the identification of possible determinants of disease occurrence.

**Analytic study:** a research investigation designed to test a hypothesis that is often used in reference to a study of an exposure-disease association.

**Association:** the extent to which the occurrence of two or more characteristics are linked either through a causal or noncausal relationship.

**Attack rate:** the proportion of persons within a population who develop a particular outcome within a specified period of time.

**Attributable risk percent:** the percentage of the overall risk of a disease outcome within exposed persons that is related to the exposure of interest.

**Beta error:** see **Type II error.**

**Bias:** a nonrandom error in a study that leads to a distorted result.

**Blinding:** assignment of treatment to individual subjects in such a way that subjects only **(single blinding)** or both subjects and treating physicians **(double blinding)** do not know the actual treatment allocation.

**Case:** a person who has a disease of interest (see also **Incident case** and **Prevalent case**).

**Case-control study:** an observational study in which subjects are sampled based on the presence (cases) or absence (controls) of the disease of interest. Information is collected about earlier exposure to risk factors of interest.

**Case fatality:** the proportion of persons with a particular disease who die from that disease within a specified period of time.

**Causality:** the extent to which the occurrence of a risk factor is responsible for the subsequent occurrence of a disease outcome.

**Clinical trial:** an experimental study that is designed to compare the therapeutic benefits of two or more treatments.

**Cluster:** a group of cases of a disease that are closely linked in time, place of occurrence, or both.

**Cohort:** a group of persons who share a common attribute, such as birth in a particular year or residence in a particular town, who are followed over time.

**Cohort study:** an observational study in which subjects are sampled based on the presence (exposed) or absence (unexposed) of a risk factor of interest. These subjects are followed over time for the development of a disease outcome of interest. (See also **Prospective cohort study** and **Retrospective cohort study**.)

**Common-source exposure:** contact with a risk factor that originates in the shared environment of multiple persons.

**Concordant results:** the same outcome status for two or more individuals, as in a pair-matched case-control study when both the case and the control are exposed (or unexposed).

**Confidence interval:** a range of values for a measure that is believed to contain the true value within a specified level (eg, 95%) of certainty.

**Confounder:** a variable that distorts the apparent relationship between an exposure and a disease of interest.

**Confounding:** a systematic error in a study that arises from mixing of the effect of the exposure of interest with other associated correlates of the disease outcome.

**Control:** in a case-control study, a subject without the disease of interest. See also **Adjustment.**

**Control group:** a population of comparison subjects in an analytic investigation.

**Correlation study:** a hypothesis-generating investigation in which the values of two or more summary characteristics are associated across different population groups.

**Cross-sectional study:** an analytic investigation in which subjects are sampled at a fixed point or period of time, and then the associations between the concurrent presence or absence of risk factors and diseases are investigated.

**Cumulative incidence:** the risk of developing a particular disease within a specified period of time.

**Death rate:** see **Mortality rate.**

**Dependent variable:** see **Outcome variable.**

**Descriptive epidemiology:** activities related to characterizing patterns of disease occurrence.

**Differential misclassification:** incorrect categorization of the status of subjects with regard to one variable (eg, exposure) that is influenced by other characteristics of interest (eg, disease status).

**Discordant results:** different outcome status for two or more individuals, as in a pair-matched case-control study when one subject in a pair is exposed and the other individual is unexposed.

**Dose-response relationship:** an exposure-disease association in which the risk of disease varies with respect to the intensity or duration of exposure.

**Ecologic fallacy:** an association between summary characteristics across populations without actual linkage of the characteristics within individual persons.

**Ecologic study:** see **Correlation study.**

**Endemic rate:** the usual rate of occurrence of particular events within a population.

**Epidemic:** a dramatic increase above the usual or expected rate of occurrence of particular events within a population.

**Epidemiology:** the study of the distribution and determinants of disease within human populations.

**Excess risk:** the extra risk of a particular disease occurring among persons exposed to a risk factor of interest. See also **Risk difference.**

**Exclusions:** persons who are eliminated from an analytic study because they do not satisfy the inclusion criteria.

**Exposure:** contact with or possession of a characteristic that is suspected to influence the risk of developing a particular disease.

**External validity:** the extent to which the conclusions of a study are correct for persons beyond those who were investigated. See also **Generalize.**

**False-negative:** a test result that is normal (negative) despite the true presence of a particular disease or a study result that incorrectly fails to identify a true effect (see also **Type II error**).

**False-positive:** a test result that is abnormal (positive) despite the true absence of the disease of interest or a study result that incorrectly indicates an effect, when in truth, the effect does not exist (see also **Type I error**).

**Follow-up study:** see **Cohort study.**

**Generalize:** the ability to extrapolate study results from the study subjects to other persons who were not investigated.

**Historical cohort study:** see **Retrospective cohort study.**

**Historical controls:** subjects in a clinical study who were previously treated with the standard therapy before the new treatment was introduced.

**Hypothesis-generating study:** an exploratory investigation designed to formulate questions that are evaluated in subsequent analytic studies.

**Hypothesis-testing study:** an analytic investigation in which one or more specific refutable suppositions is (are) evaluated.

**Incidence density:** see **Incidence rate.**

**Incidence rate:** the rapidity with which new cases of a particular disease arise within a given population.

**Incident case:** a person who is newly diagnosed with a disease of interest.

**Incubation period:** the time interval between contact with a risk factor (often an infectious agent) and the first clinical evidence of the resulting illness.

**Independent variable:** a factor that is suspected to influence the outcome of an analytic study.

**Information (or observation) bias:** a systematic error in a study that arises from the manner in which data are collected from participants.

**Intention-to-treat:** analysis of the results of a clinical trial based upon initial treatment assignment regardless of whether or not the subjects completed the full course of treatment.

**Internal validity:** the extent to which the conclusions of a study are correct for the subjects under investigation.

**Latent period:** time between exposure to a risk factor and subsequent development of clinical manifestations of a particular disease.

**Lead-time bias:** apparent increase in the length of survival with a disease as a result of earlier recognition of the disease through the use of a screening procedure.

**Length-biased sampling:** preferential detection of less aggressive forms of a disease through the use of a screening procedure.

**Matching:** a procedure for sampling comparison subjects based upon whether key attributes (ie, **matching factors**) are similar to those of subjects in the index group.

**Median survival time:** the duration from diagnosis to death that is exceeded by exactly 50% of subjects with a particular disease.

**Misclassification bias:** incorrect characterization of the status of subjects with regard to a study variable that leads to a distorted conclusion. See also **Information bias.**

**Mortality rate:** the rapidity with which persons within a given population die from a particular disease.

**Natural history:** the progression of a disease through successive stages that is often used to describe the course of an illness for which no effective treatment is available.

**Negative predictive value:** the probability that a person with a negative (normal) test result actually does not have the disease of interest.

**Nondifferential misclassification:** incorrect categorization of the status of subjects with regard to one variable (eg, exposure) that is unrelated to another characteristic of interest (eg, disease status).

**Null value:** the point on the scale of a measure of association that corresponds to no association (eg, 1 for the risk ratio and the odds ratio, and 0 for the risk difference and the attributable risk percent).

**Observation bias:** see **Information bias.**

**Observational study:** a nonexperimental analytic study in which the investigator monitors, but does not influence, the exposure status of individual subjects and their subsequent disease status.

**Odds:** the probability that a particular event will occur divided by the probability that the event will not occur.

**Odds ratio:** the odds of a particular exposure among persons with a specific disease divided by the corresponding odds of exposure among persons without the disease of interest.

**Outcome variable:** in an analytic study, the response of interest (eg, development of disease).

**Pathogen:** an agent responsible for the development of a particular disease.

**Person-time:** a unit of measurement used in the estimation of rates that reflects the amount of time observed for persons at risk of a particular event.

**Person-to-person spread:** propagation of a disease within a population by transfer from an affected person to susceptible persons.

**Placebo:** an inert substance. The **placebo effect** occurs when persons affected with a specific illness demonstrate clinical improvement upon treatment with an inert substance.

**Population at risk:** persons who are susceptible to a particular disease but who are not yet affected.

**Population-based study:** an analytic study in which subjects are sampled from the general population.

**Positive predictive value:** the probability that a person with a positive (abnormal) test result actually has the disease of interest.

**Power:** see **Statistical power.**

**Precision:** the extent to which a measurement is narrowly characterized. **Statistical precision** is inversely related to the variance of the measurement.

**Predictor variable:** see **Independent variable.**

**Prevalence:** the proportion of persons in a given population who have a particular disease at a point or interval of time.

**Prevalent case:** a person who has a disease of interest that was diagnosed in the past.

**Prospective cohort study:** a cohort study in which exposure status and subsequent occurrence of disease both occur after the onset of the investigation.

**Randomization:** procedure for assigning treatments to patients by chance.

**Rate:** the rapidity with which health events such as new diagnoses or deaths occur. See also **Incidence rate** and **Mortality rate.**

**Rate ratio:** the rate of occurrence of a specified health event among persons exposed to a particular risk factor divided by the corresponding rate among unexposed persons.

**Relative risk:** see **Risk ratio.**

**Reliability:** the extent to which multiple measurements of a characteristic are in agreement.

**Response variable:** see **Outcome variable.**

**Retrospective cohort study:** a cohort study in which exposure status and subsequent development of disease both occur prior to the onset of the investigation.

**Risk:** the probability that an event (eg, development of disease) will occur within a specific period of time.

**Risk difference:** the risk of a particular disease occurrence among persons exposed to a given risk fac-

tor minus the corresponding risk among unexposed persons.

**Risk factor:** an attribute or agent that is suspected to be related to the occurrence of a particular disease.

**Risk ratio:** the likelihood of a particular disease occurrence among persons exposed to a given risk factor divided by the corresponding likelihood among unexposed persons.

**Sample:** a subset of a target population that is chosen for investigation.

**Screening:** the use of tests to detect the presence of a particular disease among asymptomatic persons prior to the time that the disease would be recognized through routine clinical methods.

**Selection bias:** a systematic error in a study that arises from the manner in which subjects are sampled.

**Sensitivity:** the probability that a person who actually has the disease of interest will have a positive (abnormal) test result.

**Specificity:** the probability that a person who actually does not have the disease of interest will have a negative (normal) test result.

**Standardization:** an analytic procedure for obtaining a summary measure for a population by applying standard weights to the measures within subgroups of the population.

**Statistical power:** the ability of a study to detect a true effect of a specified magnitude. The statistical power corresponds to $1 -$ Type II error.

**Statistical significance:** the likelihood that a difference as large or larger than that observed between study groups could have occurred by chance alone in a sample of the size investigated. Usually, the level of statistical significance is stated as a $P$-value (eg, $P < 0.05$.)

**Surveillance:** ongoing observation of a population for rapid and accurate detection of changes in the occurrence of particular diseases.

**Survival:** the likelihood of remaining alive for a specified period of time after the diagnosis of a particular disease.

**Systematic error:** see **Bias.**

**True-negative:** a test result that is normal (negative) when the disease of interest is actually absent.

**True-positive:** a test result that is abnormal (positive) when the disease of interest is actually present.

**Type I error:** rejection of the null hypothesis when it is actually correct.

**Type II error:** failure to reject the null hypothesis when it is actually incorrect.

**Validity:** the extent to which a measurement or a study result correctly represents the characteristics or relationship of interest.

**Vital statistics:** information concerning patterns of registered life events, such as births, marriages, divorces, and deaths.

**Withdrawals:** subjects who are initially included in a study but later voluntarily or involuntarily terminate participation.

# Appendix A: Answers to Study Questions

**CHAPTER 1**

1. C
2. D
3. A
4. B
5. C
6. D
7. C
8. E
9. E
10. C

**CHAPTER 2**

1. C
2. B
3. E
4. A
5. C
6. A
7. D
8. B
9. E
10. D

**CHAPTER 3**

1. C
2. E
3. B
4. A
5. C
6. D
7. B
8. E
9. D
10. A

**CHAPTER 4**

1. D
2. B

3. E
4. A
5. C
6. B
7. D
8. E
9. A
10. C

**CHAPTER 5**

1. B
2. C
3. A
4. D
5. A
6. E
7. C
8. D
9. B
10. E

**CHAPTER 6**

1. A
2. C
3. D
4. B
5. E
6. A
7. B
8. E
9. C
10. D

**CHAPTER 7**

1. E
2. C
3. B
4. A
5. D
6. D

7. B
8. E
9. E
10. C

## CHAPTER 8

1. B
2. C
3. D
4. C
5. E
6. A
7. D
8. A
9. B
10. D

## CHAPTER 9

1. B
2. D
3. E
4. A
5. C
6. A
7. E
8. B

9. C
10. D

## CHAPTER 10

1. D
2. C
3. E
4. A
5. B
6. E
7. C
8. A
9. B
10. A

## CHAPTER 11

1. A
2. C
3. B
4. D
5. C
6. A
7. E
8. D
9. B
10. E

# Appendix B: Estimation of Sample Size Requirements for Randomized Controlled Clinical Trials

The actual formulas used to estimate sample size requirements are provided in this appendix, along with illustrative calculations from the streptokinase-tPA trial described in Chapter 7.

Prior to undertaking this study, the investigators specified an alpha level (0.05, or 5%), statistical power (90%, and thus a beta level of 10%), and the outcome difference that should be detectable (4% in LVEF). The magnitude of difference in ejection fraction was derived from a previous trial that compared LVEF in patients with acute myocardial infarction treated with or without streptokinase. The statistical comparison of LVEFs, determined prior to the study by the authors, was to be an unpaired $t$ test (see Dawson-Saunders and Trapp, 1990), which uses the mean and variance of LVEF for each group to determine whether the outcomes of the two groups are statistically different. The equation for sample size for an unpaired $t$ test is as follows:

$$n = 2 \left[ \frac{(z_\alpha - z_\beta)\sigma}{\mu_1 - \mu_2} \right]^2 \qquad (1)$$

where $n$ is the number of subjects for each treatment group, $\mu_1 - \mu_2$ is the detectable difference between the means of the two groups, $\sigma$ is the common standard deviation of each group, and $z_\alpha$ and $z_\beta$ are the values that include alpha in the two tails and beta in the lower tail of the standard normal distribution. These values can be determined from tables available in most statistical texts (see Dawson-Saunders and Trapp, 1990). The $z_\alpha$ value for a type I error of 5% is 1.96, and the $z_\beta$ value for a type II error of 10% is $-1.28$. As the acceptable level of error decreases, $z_\alpha$ and $z_\beta$ increase. In equation (1), it is assumed that the true variance for the control and treatment groups are equal. Other formulas for sample size determination are available when these variances are assumed to be different.

Note that in equation (1), the greater the absolute values of $z_\alpha$, $z_\beta$, and $\sigma$ and the smaller the difference in the means ($\mu_1 - \mu_2$), the larger the $n$, or sample size required (Table 7–2). This makes sense intu-itively, since smaller differences in means between groups would be harder to detect, and greater variability within the groups would tend to blur inter-group differences. To decrease the probability that one would make a type I or type II error would also require a larger number of observations (ie, a larger sample size).

For the streptokinase-tPA study, the investigators estimated that the mean LVEF for the streptokinase group would be 58% (0.58), and they wanted the study to be able to detect a difference in LVEF of 4% (0.04) between the streptokinase and tPA groups. The standard deviation for the two groups was estimated to be 0.105 from previous studies and assumed to be equal for the two groups. Therefore, the sample size for each group was calculated using equation (1):

$$n = 2 \left[ \frac{(1.96 + 1.28)\, 0.105}{(0.62 - 0.58)} \right]^2$$

and $n = 145$. Because the total sample size required to obtain a power of 90% was 145 in each group, a total of 290 subjects was needed. Restated: If the true difference in mean LVEFs is 4% or greater, then the probability that the researchers will find no difference between the mean LVEFs of the streptokinase and tPA groups with an equally divided sample size of 290 is only 10%.

If death within 6 months had been chosen as the primary end point for this study, the required sample size could have been determined on the basis of the proportion of patients who would die within 6 months after infarction, using the following equation:

$$n = \left[ \frac{z_\alpha \sqrt{2\pi_c(1 - \pi_c)} - z_\beta \sqrt{\pi_t(1 - \pi_t) + \pi_c(1 - \pi_c)}}{\pi_t - \pi_c} \right]^2$$

where $\pi_c$ and $\pi_t$ are the proportion of patients who will die within 6 months in the control (streptokinase) group and the treatment group (tPA), respectively, and $z_\alpha$ and $z_\beta$ have the same meaning as in equation (1).

Again, without memorizing this formula, we can intuitively understand how its various components contribute to sample size. The larger the $z_\alpha$ and $z_\beta$—ie, the smaller the acceptable type I and type II errors—the larger the sample size required; and the smaller the difference in $\pi_c$ and $\pi_t$, the larger the sample size required. What may not be so intuitively obvious is the relation of sample size to the distance of $\pi_c$ from 0.5. The part of the equation $\pi_c(1 - \pi_c)$ is maximized, and therefore the numerator is greater, when $\pi_c = 0.5$. Movement of $\pi_c$ away from 0.5 reduces the required sample size.

If one expected the proportion dying in the streptokinase group to be 0.10 and wanted to be able to detect a reduction of mortality from 0.10 to 0.05 using tPA, then the sample size would be calculated as follows:

$$n = \left[ \frac{1}{(0.05 - 0.10)} \left\{ 1.96 \sqrt{2 \times 0.10 \times 0.90} - (-1.28) \sqrt{(0.05 \times 0.95) + (0.10 \times 0.90)} \right\} \right]^2$$

and $n = 683$. Therefore, a total of 1366 subjects equally divided between groups would be required to answer the question, "Is there a reduction in mortality from 10% to 5% using tPA instead of streptokinase?" The researchers for the streptokinase-tPA study may have felt that this was the most important question but did not feel that they could recruit this many patients in a timely manner. By measuring LVEF—a known predictor of mortality—the researchers were able to recruit enough patients in a reasonable amount of time to answer a relevant and clinically important question.

# Appendix C: Method for Determining the Confidence Interval Around the Risk Ratio

An approximate 95% confidence interval ($CI$) around the point estimate of the risk ratio ($RR$) can be calculated using the following formula:

**95% $CI$**

$$= (RR) \exp\left[\pm 1.96 \sqrt{VAR(\ln RR)}\right]$$

**where**

$$\sqrt{VAR(\ln RR)}$$

$$= \sqrt{\frac{1 - A/(A + C)}{A} + \frac{1 - B/(B + D)}{B}}$$

where exp is the base of the natural logarithm raised to the quantity within the brackets and $A$, $B$, $C$, and $D$ represent the numerical entries in the summary format in Table 8–6 and VAR($\ln RR$) is the estimated variance of the natural logarithm of the RR. This confidence interval is approximate because it is based on a computational short-cut for estimating the variance of the natural logarithm of the $RR$. For relatively large samples, this approximation yields confidence limits that are quite close to the exact values, which are much more difficult to calculate.

The 95% $CI$ for the 10-minute Apgar score (0–3 versus 4–6) relationship to infant mortality described in Chapter 8 is:

**95% $CI$**

$$= (2.8) \exp\left[\pm 1.96 \sqrt{\frac{(1 - 0.344)}{42} + \frac{(1 - 0.125)}{43}}\right]$$

$$= (2.8) \exp\left[\pm 1.96 \sqrt{0.0156 + 0.0203}\right]$$

$$= (2.8) \exp(\pm 0.37)$$

**Lower bound** $= (2.8) \exp(-0.37) = 1.9$

**Upper bound** $= (2.8) \exp(+0.37) = 4.1$

# Appendix D: Method for Determining the Confidence Interval Around the Odds Ratio

An approximate 95% confidence interval $(CI)$ around the point estimate of the $OR$ for an unmatched case-control study can be calculated using the following formula:

$$95\% \; CI = (OR) \exp \left[ \pm 1.96 \sqrt{\frac{1}{A} + \frac{1}{B} + \frac{1}{C} + \frac{1}{D}} \right]$$

where exp is the base of the natural logarithm raised to the quantity in the brackets, and $A$, $B$, $C$, and $D$ represent the numerical entries into the summary format in Table 9–4. This confidence interval is approximate because it is based upon a computational shortcut to estimating the variance of the natural logarithm of the $OR$. For relatively large sample sizes, this approximation yields confidence bounds that are quite close to the exact values, which are much more difficult to calculate.

For the data in Table 9–5 relating aspirin use to Reye's syndrome in a hypothetical unmatched case-control study, the 95% $CI$ was calculated as follows:

$$95\% \; CI = (10.2) \exp \left[ \pm 1.96 \sqrt{\frac{1}{190} + \frac{1}{10} + \frac{1}{130} + \frac{1}{70}} \right]$$

$$= (10.2) \; \textbf{exp} \; [\pm \; 0.70]$$

Lower bound $= (10.2) \; \textbf{exp} \; [-0.70] = 5.1$

Upper bound $= (10.2) \; \textbf{exp} \; [+0.70] = 20.5$

Similarly, an approximate 95% $CI$ around the point estimate of an $OR$ from a pair-matched case-control study can be calculated using the following formula:

$$95\% \; CI = (OR) \exp \left[ \pm 1.96 \sqrt{\frac{1}{X} + \frac{1}{Y}} \right]$$

where exp is the base of the natural logarithm raised to the quantity in the brackets, and $X$ and $Y$ represent the numerical entries in the summary format in Table 9–6.

For the data in Table 9–7 relating aspirin use to Reye's syndrome in a hypothetical pair-matched case-control study, the 95% $CI$ was calculated as follows:

$$95\% \; CI = (11.4) \exp \left[ \pm 1.96 \sqrt{\frac{1}{57} + \frac{1}{5}} \right]$$

$$= (11.4) \; \textbf{exp} \; [\pm \; 0.91]$$

Lower bound $= (11.4) \; \textbf{exp} \; [-0.91] = 4.6$

Upper bound $= (11.4) \; \textbf{exp} \; [+0.91] = 28.3$

# Index

NOTE: A *t* following a page number indicates tabular material and an *f* following a page number indicates a figure.

## Basic Science Textbooks

*Jawetz, Melnick & Adelberg's*
**Medical Microbiology, 19/e**
*Brooks, Butel & Ornston*
1991, ISBN 0-8385-6241-8, A6241-2
**Concise Pathology**
*Chandrasoma & Taylor*
1991, ISBN 0-8385-1320-4, A1320-9
**Correlative Neuroanatomy, 21/e**
*deGroot & Chusid*
1991, ISBN 0-8385-1332-8, A1332-4
**Review of Medical Physiology, 15/e**
*Ganong*
1991, ISBN 0-8385-8418-7, A8418-4
**Physiology: A Study Guide, 3/e**
*Ganong*
1989, ISBN 0-8385-7875-6, A7875-6
**Basic Histology, 7/e**
*Junqueira, Carniero & Kelly*
1992, ISBN 0-8385-0576-7, A0576-7
**Basic & Clinical Pharmacology, 5/e**
*Katzung*
1992, ISBN 0-8385-0562-7, A0562-7
**Pharmacology: Examination & Review, 3/e**
*Katzung & Trevor*
1992, ISBN 0-8385-7807-1, A7807-9
**Medical Microbiology & Immunology**
*Examination & Board Review, 2/e*
*Levinson & Jawetz*
1991, ISBN 0-8385-6262-0, A6262-8
**Harper's Biochemistry, 22/e**
*Murray, et al.*
1991, ISBN 0-8385-3640-9, A3640-8
**Basic Histology**
*Examination & Board Review, 2/e*
*Paulsen*
1992, ISBN 0-8385-0569-4, A0569-2
**Basic & Clinical Immunology, 7/e**
*Stites & Terr*
1991, ISBN 0-8385-0544-9, A0544-5
**Basic Human Immunology**
*Stites & Terr*
1991, ISBN 0-8385-0543-0, A0543-7

## Clinical Science Textbooks

**Fluid & Electrolytes**
*Physiology & Pathophysiology*
*Cogan*
1991, ISBN 0-8385-2546-6, A2546-8
**Basic and Clinical Biostatistics**
*Dawson-Saunders & Trapp*
1990, ISBN 0-8385-6200-0, A6200-8
**Review of General Psychiatry, 3/e**
*Goldman*
1992, ISBN 0-8385-8428-4, A8428-3
**Principles of Clinical Electrocardiography, 13/e**
*Goldschlager & Goldman*
1989, ISBN 0-8385-7951-5, A7951-5

**Basic and Clinical Endocrinology, 3/e**
*Greenspan*
1990, ISBN 0-8385-0545-7, A0545-2
**Occupational Medicine**
*LaDou*
1990, ISBN 0-8385-7207-3, A7207-2
**Clinical Anatomy**
*Lindner*
1989, ISBN 0-8385-1259-3, A1259-9
**Clinical Anesthesiology**
*Morgan & Mikhail*
1992, ISBN 0-8385-1324-7, A1324-1
**Dermatology**
*Orkin, Maibach & Dahl*
1991, ISBN 0-8385-1288-7, A1288-8
**Clinical Neurology, 2/e**
*Simon, Aminoff & Greenberg*
1992, ISBN 0-8385-1311-5, A1311-8
**Clinical Cardiology, 5/e**
*Sokolow, McIlroy & Cheitlin*
1990, ISBN 0-8385-1266-6, A1266-4
**Clinical Thinking in Surgery**
*Sterns*
1988, ISBN 0-8385-5686-8, A5686-9
**Smith's General Urology, 13/e**
*Tanagho & McAninch*
1992, ISBN 0-8385-8608-2, A8608-0
**General Ophthalmology, 13/e**
*Vaughan, Asbury & Riordan-Eva*
1992, ISBN 0-8385-3115-6, A3115-1

## CURRENT Clinical References

**CURRENT Pediatric Diagnosis & Treatment, 11/e**
*Hathaway, et al.*
1992, ISBN 0-8385-1440-5, A1440-5
**CURRENT Obstetric & Gynecologic Diagnosis & Treatment, 7/e**
*Pernoll*
1991, ISBN 0-8385-1424-3, A1424-9
**CURRENT Emergency Diagnosis & Treatment, 4/e**
*Saunders & Ho*
1992, ISBN 0-8385-1347-6, A1347-2
**CURRENT Medical Diagnosis & Treatment 1992, 31/e**
*Schroeder, et al.*
1992, ISBN 0-8385-1438-3, A1438-9
**CURRENT Surgical Diagnosis & Treatment, 9/e**
*Way*
1991, ISBN 0-8385-1426-X, A1426-4

---

*Order information on reverse.*

---

## LANGE Clinical Manuals

**Dermatology**
*Diagnosis and Therapy*
*Bondi, Jegasothy & Lazarus*
1990, ISBN 0-8385-1274-7, A1274-8
**Office & Bedside Procedures**
*Chesnutt & Dewar*
1992, ISBN 0-8385-1095-7, A1095-7
**Psychiatry**
*Diagnosis & Treatment, 2/e*
*Flaherty, Davis & Janicak*
1992, ISBN 0-8385-1267-4, A1267-2
**Neonatology**
*Management, Procedures, On-Call Problems, Diseases, Drugs, 2/e*
*Gomella*
1992, ISBN 0-8385-1284-4, A1284-7
**Clinician's Pocket Reference, 6/e**
*Gomella*
1989, ISBN 0-8385-1212-7, A1212-8
**Drug Therapy, 2/e**
*Katzung*
1991, ISBN 0-8385-1312-3, A1312-6
**Poisoning and Drug Overdose**
*Olson*
1990, ISBN 0-8385-1297-6, A1297-9
**Ambulatory Medicine**
*Primary Care of Families*
*Schwiebert & Mengle*
1992, ISBN 0-8385-1294-1, A1294-6
**Internal Medicine**
*Diagnosis and Therapy, 2/e*
*Stein*
1991, ISBN 0-8385-1299-2, A1299-5
**Surgery**
*Diagnosis & Therapy*
*Stillman*
1989, ISBN 0-8385-1283-6, A1283-9
**Medical Perioperative Management**
*Wolfsthal*
1989, ISBN 0-8385-1298-4, A1298-7

## LANGE Handbooks

**Handbook of Gynecology & Obstetrics**
*Brown & Crombleholme*
1992, ISBN 0-8385-3608-5, A3608-5
**Handbook of Clinical Endocrinology, 2/e**
*Fitzgerald*
1991, ISBN 0-8385-3615-8, A3615-0
*Silver, Kempe, Bruyn & Fulginiti's*
**Handbook of Pediatrics, 16/e**
*Merenstein, Kaplan & Rosenberg*
1991, ISBN 0-8385-3639-5, A3639-0
**Pocket Guide to Commonly Prescribed Drugs**
*Levine*
1992, ISBN 0-8385-8023-8, A8023-2
**Pocket Guide to Diagnostic Tests**
*Detmer, et al.*
1992, ISBN 0-8385-8020-3, A8020-8

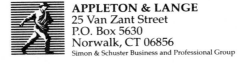